# THE BIG SHIFT

## Build Your Own Economy, Fire Your Boss ... and Walk Out Laughing!

Ian D. Billingham

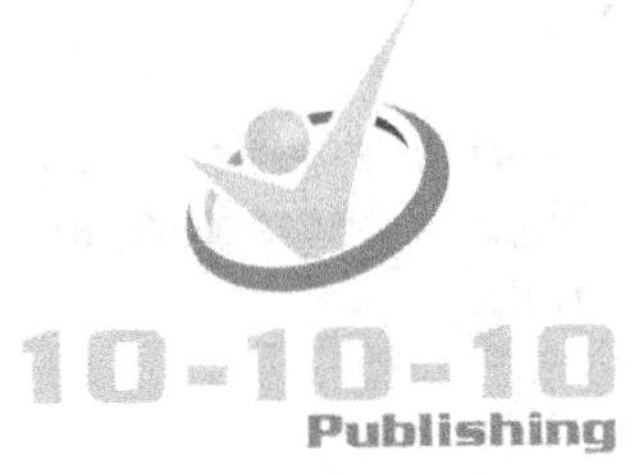

The Big Shift: Build Your Own Economy, Fire Your Boss...and Walk Out Laughing!
www.MakeTheBigShiftBook.com



Published By
10-10-10 Publishing
200-455 Apple Creek Blvd.
Markham, Ontario  L3R 9X7

First 10-10-10 Publishing Paperback Edition (September, 2019)

# TABLE OF CONTENTS

*This book is dedicated to God's grace and mercy,
and to the second chance for the human spirit in the pursuit of
freedom, opportunity, prosperity, and love.*

# FOREWORD

*The Big Shift,* by Ian Billingham, addresses what is likely to be the most important topic of change that is impacting you and your loved ones on a deep physical, emotional and spiritual level. The system of upbringing and society has molded you in the traditional way of earning a living, and forcing you to work harder than ever just to keep your head above water, than to confront and deal with the massive shift that has already happened in the modern economy around you. You are imprisoned by your own thinking and the traditional way of earning a living; and yet, you're in the golden age of freedom and opportunity.

So, when Ian approached me with a synopsis of what he wanted to write about, I just knew you needed to hear more of what he has to say. That's why I was so excited to endorse Ian's book as he lays out the shift that is invisibly impacting you right before your eyes...and offers a serious alternative that you need to hear.

Ian gets right into it in chapter one as he sets the stage with his own corporate walk of shame out the door in a way you can imagine it happening to you. Ian is just your average guy with a middle-class upbringing, molded and pushed into getting good grades, a piece of paper from a reputable college in exchange for the illusion of a lifetime guarantee of financial security and living *happily ever after.* Job redundancy and frustration has become the norm. Ian thought it could never happen to him and yet it did. And so it can happen to you too.

In *The Big Shift,* Ian is literally giving you his 20/20 hindsight of what you need to start doing right now instead of dreading each day in a job you know you already hate, heading towards an insecure future, and the almost certainty of imminent job redundancy. Consider his book a look into a version of a possible future you. He's handing it to you on a silver platter, how even you can prepare yourself for the biggest shift you need to make in your life towards living the rest of it in abundance, and avoiding the shock and desperation of where that will leave you if you don't.

This book is a warning, but it's also one of hope and opportunity, as Ian's experience of success and failure is laid out raw for you to avoid the traps you may be heading into, so that you can take the good stuff straight to the bank. It's written as if Ian is sitting down in a coffee shop and speaking candidly to you about the current future you're heading into, but it also provides unique battle-proven insights and practical advice on how you can start crafting an alternative future for yourself right now.

Ian is the consummate professional, a great communicator and has a very clear and concise way of compressing complex, interconnected ideas of the new age business world, into simple need-to-know building blocks that you can start applying now in building a life of independence, financial freedom, and a lifestyle you and your family have been dreaming about.

I congratulate you on getting a copy of this book, and in making *The Big Shift* forward.

**Raymond Aaron**
**New York Times Bestselling Author**

# ACKNOWLEDGEMENTS

It was a challenge to start to put pen to paper for my acknowledgement of the innumerable people who have made an impact and have influenced my journey in business, in life, understanding myself, revealing my own faults, learning to love, and the continuing desire to be a better version of me today than I was yesterday.

To my wife, partner in life, lover, and soul mate, **Susy**, who has stood by me through the amazingly good times, and the lows, who inspired me with her amazing positivity and magnetic energy, and who has taught me how to love. And to my kids, **Mike** and **Yasmin,** who are the inspiration for why I do what I do, as they head into an exciting future of opportunity in moving the world in pictures and film, impacting and inspiring youngsters around the world.

To my dad, **Nico**, who instilled in me the values of fatherhood, and who taught me the appreciation of words (even though it didn't sink in until 40-some years later!); and to my mom, **Sylvia,** who has supported each step of my career, and for our conversations throughout life. My big sis, **Sharon,** with her amazing intellect, becoming the first person in the family to have published a book; and my bro, the first doctor in the Billingham clan, Dr. **Simon,** whose heart and passion for healing others is a true inspiration to us all.

To **Eric Worre** and his numerous words of wisdom, and his video presence, amazing teaching philosophy, and ground-breaking documentary, *Rise of the Entrepreneur*; and of course, his awarding-winning book, *Go Pro,* which inspired me and millions the world over in my early days in getting started as an entrepreneur. Eric, I was privileged to have finally met you, in Austria, in 2015—thank you for what you continue to do.

I want to extend my gratitude to **Bernard D. Evans,** for revealing the greater perspective of my business and my talents, and how to serve the marketplace with my skills, and for his mentorship on my journey in faith, shaping my character in attitude to walk in discernment and in truth, and in discovering my greater plan and purpose in life.

**Ray Higdon** is not only a rock star in my books, but his entertaining method of teaching and products got me started with on-line branding. The most impactful teaching was his simple method of self-introduction, story-telling, and vlogging, which inspired me toward creating over 160 videos in less than 6 months, from which I've also been able to teach thousands, the world over, with my own 4-step process that I've included in this book—I look forward to the day that we meet, so I can shake your hand.

A true legend, and inspiration to my own speaking career, **Tony Robbins**, whose abundant energy and superhuman positive energy inspired my wife and I to walk on fire at UPW-London, April 2017, and for our (my wife's, in fact) face-to-face encounter, in front of 10,000+ people.

**Pip Stelnik** was such a terrific, entertaining, engaging, and knowledgeable trainer on property when we attended a workshop in Hong Kong, hosted by him. He made a big impact on my career in becoming an international seminar speaker and educator.

**Robert Kiyosaki,** you have shifted my overall approach and concept of money, and you've become a welcomed guest in our home, through your videos, books, and seminars.

**Ryan Daniel,** for our trusted partnership, and for your amazing technical acumen on funnels and advertising; it was a tremendous ride, and I look forward to our continued collaboration.

To your generous giving and secrets-sharing, **Shaqir Hussein,** you instilled in me the art and science from the stage of story-telling, humor, and energy. I am in deep gratitude to you for giving my son, Mike, his first filming break, and for taking him to see the world.

To **Chris Rowell**, a legend in selling, and in managing diverse and remote events teams internationally, who taught me the greater role of a seminar speaker, with becoming the CEO of the room.

To the team of rock stars that I toured with on the road, and the unforgettable experiences and *shenanigans*—**Angela Barrows, Amilia Murad, Abraham Premean, Ben Sweet, Carl Kapapiro, Emilia Pisano, Humayun Miah, James Collier, Kalpna Suthar, Khalid Miah, Liyana Kemissi, Martin Arul, Michelle MacFarlane, Michelle Yong, Marita Teigland, Nicola Raft, Nora Kelmendi, Roger Daniel Raju, Sean Wray, Shylvera Teo, Stefan Fincis, and Vas Babeiu**—you all taught me teamwork, closing, and how to LMAO again!!

**Hayley Andrews,** who spent 4 days with my wife and me, so patiently offloading everything she knew about property investing in the UK. She consulted with us and mapped out a long-term strategy plan for our property portfolio plan. She was such a terrific mentor, on top of being a major property player, and gave us such honest and constructive feedback on our investment strategy.

**Steve Gibson, Sam Gibson, and Dave Pawan,** of Carlson Gracie Surrey, for their dedication to changing people's lives through the art of Brazilian *Jiu-Jitsu,* and for their instrumental roles in my own journey of becoming a humble student in life again. There's nothing more focused on solving a problem in life than when you're being thrown around by a skilled *jiu-jitsu* practitioner.

# Chapter 1

# Flippin' Burgers

*"The most difficult thing is the decision to act; the rest is merely tenacity. The fears are paper tigers. You can do anything you decide to do. You can act to change and control your life; and the procedure, the process is its own reward."*
– Amelia Earhart

## Tied with "Silken Handcuffs"

The 40/40 plan is over. Working that 40-hour week for the next 40 years, and expecting to live happily ever after, is a fairy tale that has turned into a nightmare. The notion of job security started disappearing in late 1989, when Sir Tim Berners-Lee established a communication link between a Hypertext Transfer Protocol (HTTP) and a server through the internet, which became the precursor to the World Wide Web as we know it today. That was when we entered the Internet Age. Technology has changed everything, including what it means to earn a living.

You're only still in a job because the company hasn't figured out how to outsource it...yet.

You're working even harder than you did last year, because *they*, the company, decided to let go a bunch of your colleagues, so now you get to work double time. Your bank account, however, doesn't say anything different.

I remember, way back in the 1980s (and I can't believe I just said *way back in the 80s!!*), when I was working at McDonald's. It was during a time when I was still flipping burgers over a hot grill, and when the burgers still had taste.

Growing up in Hong Kong, I was working full, 10-hour shifts, at what was then the second biggest McDonald's outlet in the world. The biggest one was just further down toward the harbor, in Star Ferry Terminal.

I loved working there. We had about as much staff behind the counter as there were customers in the restaurant. It was crazy. We were split into several strategic team units, all carefully choreographed to serve up the customer's order in 30 seconds or less.

I'm a mixed-race kid:  Dad is English; Mom's Chinese. I stuck out like a sore thumb in Hong Kong, among a sea of black-haired Chinese. I was unique, and my entire staff wanted to get to know me better because I had that exotic look of a Eurasian kid, and I spoke fluent Cantonese. I had fun with everybody. I eventually quit because my four-foot short shift supervisor couldn't stand the attention I was getting, and she started dishing out *BS* tasks. Everyone knew what was going on.

It was a *power play* by the senior rank.

Fast forward 30 years, and the burgers taste like plastic. Gone are the days of grills and the smoky barbecue fragrance from the back kitchen.  Self-serving kiosks have replaced at least half the staff now in any McDonald's restaurant that you'll find anywhere in the world.

This is one example to illustrate what's happening on a global, macro level. And it's happening at an exponential rate, no matter the industry.

We're in the age of exponential growth. Big data is now dictating how computers are already transforming the workplace, replacing human beings. Never in our history has our way of life been challenged so profoundly. Gone are the days of earning an honest day's work to put food on the table and a shelter over our heads—the secure thought of being taken care of for the rest of our lives is obsolete. We are being replaced by artificial intelligence and robots, and if you think you're in a career where no non-human system can ever replace you...think again.

Someone just turned the speed dial up on the treadmill, and now you're frantically racing against time just to keep that paycheck coming in. The traditional workplace has caused a tremendous human imbalance in our spirit. As you head to work in frustration, you lack fulfillment, because the value you put into the workplace is not equally being matched in return.

No company will ever pay you what you're truly worth. Companies just can't afford to do that anymore.

It's the share price that the boys in the boardroom are obsessed about. Global expansion into new markets has become more challenging. The great promise of Southeast Asia, from the late 80s, didn't move the dial much, as social economic progress has been stagnant. Japan seems to have accepted stagnation as a new way of life since the bubble burst in the early 1990s. The great hope in China, for growth, is over for Western companies, as homebred Chinese enterprises are dominating the most populous country in the world...and they're looking for global domination. You can't get much growth out of Russia these days, because the heydays of double-digit growth, driven by distribution expansion from Moscow to Vladivostok, is tapped out.

I worked in Russia, for 3 years, for a big tobacco company, just about the time when crazy growth numbers were starting to slow down because the company had effectively maximized distribution expansion across the Federation. There was pressure on organic growth, and life in the office got very intense and stressful. It was like sitting in a sauna, and somebody else just turned up the temperature, and you're literally suffocating with no way out.

"You're tied with silken handcuffs," my dad would always say to me. I fell out of love with the career I had chosen, and life was starting to get small. It was about survival. Nothing was stopping me from leaving, but the need of a paycheck to provide for the family was the yoke I was shouldering. The money was good and kept me imprisoned. The alternative was just unthinkable.

Quitting? Starting my own business? Being an entrepreneur? Yeah, right!

## Letting Go of Getting Let Go

I spent 23 years in corporate. Eighteen of those, I gave my loyal blood to one company, at a time when company loyalty was highly regarded. Even though the career had its perks of global travel and living in different cultures, you tend to become myopic in your view of the world when working for someone for so long. I worked in big tobacco for such a long time that everything about my life revolved around cigarettes. I was programmed into constantly thinking about how to sell more.

Well, all that changed almost overnight.

I got the message on Friday, January 13, 2012, at the Copacabana Beach Hotel, in Rio de Janeiro. My wife, Susy, and I were taking some much needed downtime. January was the typical time of year for employee performance assessments and appraisals, to figure out the salary increases and bonuses that were due out in April.

The text read, "Ian, we have a problem." My heart just sank. I knew what my boss was referring to. The impending news was just too much, on top of an already stressful situation my wife and I were in.

You see, I got the message exactly seven days before my wife was due for urgent, major surgery to remove a massive tumor from her breast. She had been diagnosed with breast cancer a couple of months earlier.

Susy got through the eight-hour surgery fine. I remained with her in Brazil, and put our daughter into a new school. After about a month, when she was strong enough to get up and about and start her radiology, I had to return home to Croatia, where we were living at the time, to figure things out.

In the following nine months, my wife was fighting for her life — and I was seven thousand miles away, fighting for our livelihood.

I worked my tail off and not only achieved some terrific results in the business, but I was almost single-handedly leading a project that would restructure a multi-country regional business into independent, autonomous organisations…and eliminate my job in the process.

Susy went through radiology and chemo treatment miraculously smoothly; she didn't lose a single strand of hair. It was a miracle. A few years later, she went on to write and publish her first book, *Be Your Own Miracle;* and today, she's an international speaker and mind trainer, teaching others around the world the techniques of overcoming life's challenges, from her experience and what she had to go through.

We were finally reunited, but the company had already set in motion a different plan for me. My time was up. Whatever I had achieved at work in those last twelve months, was just not enough to shift the tide in my favor.

I was on my way out, but as a last, blatant act of covering their ass, the company did propose to send me to look after Pakistan and Afghanistan. That's how sneaky they were.

Susy and my daughter had already returned back to Croatia, in time for the news. That night, Susy and I spoke at length over at least one bottle of wine (might have been more, but it's all still a blur), and agreed on the decision. Never would I let anyone do that to me and my family again. I would never allow myself to be dependent on anyone else dictating my fate…ever.

The next morning, I marched into the office of HR and told them to draw up the papers. Their reaction was one of shock, but I was ready. Eighteen years of loyalty, and it all ended rather unceremoniously.

The liberation I felt was unbelievable. It was a feeling that was so foreign and forgotten, yet so familiar, as if it were a God-given right for every human being to be free. I was only free when I chose to let go of being let go. It was time to move on to the next exciting chapter of my life.

We took it easy for the following two months as we prepared to head back to Hong Kong. But I could never have prepared myself for the shock that was awaiting me.

## Your True Worth Is Inside You

When you've been in a dark tunnel for so long, it takes quite some time for your eyes to adjust as you emerge into the light. I was now free to pursue a new career in the light of opportunity. It's just amazing, when you've been doing something for so long for one company, how your life revolves around a singular plane—your brain; your Blackberry or iPhone, shackling you to your company email server; your social circle—and it was all centered around *the company*.

After 8 months of looking for a job, the market determined that I was overqualified, unemployable, and irrelevant. The world I emerged back into had completely shifted.

Today, company organisations are getting flatter to save costs; there are fewer and fewer jobs at the senior level, and there is much more intense competition for candidates applying for the few jobs that are available. Although there are more jobs being created, most of these only rely on specialized skills, which seem so generic and commoditized that anyone lucky enough to be accepted will only face the inevitability of being expendable. It's an employer's market now. Companies can suppress salaries because there is in fact an oversupply of skilled talent out there. Hiring managers are also not about to take the risk of deciding outside the established cookie-cutter approach to profiling and hiring senior executives.

At 43 years old, I was stuck!

I did, however, have all this free time on my hands. It was great. I regained so much lost time with the family, and I was able to attend all my daughter's school events. We even went on vacation to Thailand, just Yasmin and me, when her mom had to head back to Brazil, briefly for her regular check-ups.

The biggest wake-up call was that I had to reinvent and reinvest in my knowledge of a changed world, and learn about the alternative careers out there that rose out of this massive shift in the economy.

I was about to enter the world of the entrepreneur...but I didn't know it yet.

The average person stops investing in their adult education after the age of twenty-three, believing that the college degree would set them up for life, and that the company would invest in their development, and take care of them up to and after retirement. What the average person actually ends up doing, is surrendering the rest of their lives to a system that's already broken.

Over the years, I've started, and shut down, several other different successful businesses. For over twenty years, I knew how to run companies for somebody else; but I had no clue how to start one myself. This only came about because I invested heavily into my education, unlearning and retraining my brain away from an employee mentality, into one filled with the entrepreneurial spirit, and a mindset of abundance, persistence, and tenacity.

You need to realise and start internalizing, in your spirit and soul, that your true worth can only be manifested on your terms, and not by anyone or any company who is only prepared to pay you at the market rate—don't be like corn. You have way more value to send out into the marketplace than to continue trading your time for money.

## You Need to Buy Your Time Back

Back in 2015, I tagged along with a good friend of mine, who wanted to drag me to an event about marketing and business. I really had no idea, but I had time on my hands, and I thought, *what the heck.*

I had never been to one of these events before. It was in a hotel conference room, and when we arrived, about a hundred or so people were hanging around outside. There was definitely a buzz of anticipation and excitement in the air. We were eventually allowed inside the conference room, and little did I know, my life was about to change.

The speaker was speaking my language. He was talking about what I had spent the last 2 years researching and discovering: The world has changed, job security is out the window, and technology has opened up the golden era of opportunity and new business start-ups. Flashes of big-name, successful entrepreneurs, that the speaker personally knew, blew up on the big screen. He went on to reveal that it is not raw academic intellect that makes these people successful, but investing in yourself and doing something about what you already know...and taking action.

It all made sense...but I didn't know how it was relevant to me. Then, all of a sudden, out came that phrase that I'll never forget: *"You need a system that will buy your time back."* Everything else darkened, and it seemed like a spotlight came out from nowhere and beamed directly on the speaker. I felt as though I were the only person in the room, and the speaker was talking not just to me but *through* me.

Employees earn a paycheck by showing up at the office and trading their time for money. Even if you work for yourself, like running a restaurant, or you're a doctor or lawyer, you're still charging out your time, and your business can't function or grow without you showing up. Working for yourself is essentially owning your own job.

What true entrepreneurs do is that they look for or create systems that generate cash-flow, independent of you showing up to work. You need a business to work on, not in.

I found this absolutely intriguing and fascinating, so I made a decision that day; and I have since spent my last few years leveraging systems, and building my own, and teaching other business start-ups and entrepreneurs how to do the same.

I don't take on any clients who have the misconception that starting your own business is easy.

It takes years to build out a system that works with proven product ideas and services that the marketplace wants, and customers that keep coming back and paying you lots of money to solve their problems. A business only exists if it comes up with a solution to a customer problem. Entrepreneurs are problem solvers. Entrepreneurship is the result of years of grinding it out.

You're working hard in your job anyway, so why not start directing some of that energy and focus into building something longer term. You will be surprised to hear that starting your own business, in the new economy, is actually a better, more secure way.

And that's *the big shift* you're going to have to make.

## Harnessing the Power of Technology

I watched an interview with Paul Zane Pilzer (who's a really big deal!), who said that those who can harness the power of technology, and leverage it to their advantage, will become the rich class of the 21st century.

Now, this sounded like a bunch of hype when I first heard him say that. But it's true. So let me break that down logically so that it makes sense to you.

In the old days, businesses could only grow and expand if you opened up another store, invested in more employees and training, more trucks on the street, and more inventory in your warehouse. Before you could even begin to generate more sales revenue, you had to sink a whole lot of capital into the business.

In today's world, the odds of you going out of business in six months, with this kind of brick-and-mortar model, are stacked against you. You'll have better odds at the casino than trying to build a traditional physical business.

Growing and scaling your business today, through technology, eliminates all these headaches.

It works best when you have a digital product or service, because you can deliver and fulfill that product to your customer anywhere in the world, without the need of physical inventory or shipping costs. It's instant and it's digital. Whether you're selling t-shirts, mugs, or any other consumer product, you can source it from China, never have to touch the inventory, and it'll get fulfilled directly to your end customer. That's called *drop-shipping*. Expand your business? Just open up your business website to new countries, instantly.

No more trucks, employees, or inventory.

Your accountant now lives in the cloud, via cloud-accounting software like QuickBooks or Xero; your designers live in India, and you can get Madison Avenue-level creative quality in a matter of days...for just a few bucks, that's Fiverr. Finding products in your e-commerce store, and having orders from China pushed to your customers anywhere in the world, couldn't be simpler than using the Oberlo app; and your funnels (we'll get into that later in the book), email marketing campaigns, sales, fulfillment, and customer support can all now be done with powerfully sophisticated yet easy-to-use, drag-and-drop software, without the traditional heavy costs of hiring employees and staff that do nothing but complain.

Every single operational and repetitive procedure can now be outsourced into systems and software apps that just make starting a business in the new economy so much simpler. This enables you to remove all the heavy operating costs from your business so that you can focus on your company's creativity, product innovation, and marketing—the true role of the entrepreneur—keeping more profits down in your bottom line.

Application software, or apps, are like the employees in your organisation. Apps deal with the day-to-day operations of your business, which just gets things moving along. Instead of heavy monthly salaries, and employee benefits and taxes that can drain your cash flow, get your hands on some apps and third party software for just a few bucks a month for a subscription. They make your business run smoothly and seamlessly. Or you can deal with staff, morale, and politics, and vacations that create unnecessary disruptions in your business.

Most amateur *wannabes* complain about the costs of doing business: You need this software, and that subscription, and you have to pay for this and pay for that. When you're in a job, you don't have to worry about these costs. It's when you have to pay for them out of your own pocket for your business that it really starts to get to you, because you've never been a business owner before.

It's amazing when I teach startup entrepreneurs the list of things that they need to set up and pay for if they want a twenty-first century business that's future-proof. I get a lot of push back and negative vibes that tells me they don't get it. I have a simple response when challenged. You can pay the $49 a month subscription for the software, or $2,000 for a physical person to do that for you. Which one would you choose?

Remember: Apps and software are the employee robots of your business.

## Your True Wealth Is Your Time

The reason I wrote this book stemmed from the pain, dissatisfaction, lack of fulfillment, and *lies* of the corporate job career, and the realization of seeing this widespread problem trend all over the world. I wasn't just an isolated, unfortunate victim. It's happening all around us today.

But more importantly, the book is about hope.

*The Big Shift* is a dedication to those who want more out of life — to those who want to change the world, and to those who want freedom; and to you who want more meaning in your life, to live out your purpose and calling.

I thought to myself, if more and more people around the world are feeling disenfranchised with their job or career, they're never going to shift and do something about it, and get out of the *rat race,* until the proverbial s*** hits the fan.

I wrote this book to you as my 20/20 hindsight for your future. What if I could help you see what you're heading toward, and inspire you to start something now, and avoid the pain and panic later down the road when you're up against a financial life challenge?

So, I'm going to teach you some fundamental core habits, behaviours, and skills to prepare you to build a business around what you already know and are passionate about.

I'm going to take you through a sequential flow that you should follow in order to embark on your journey. There is the psychology and the emotions of the entrepreneur, which if you don't understand, and don't confront and fix it within yourself, you're going to have a really hard time.

I'll share the foundational building blocks of what you need to have in place in building your empire. I'll steer you away from the traps I fell into, which just about every entrepreneur does, so that it can save you a lot of time and a lot of money in getting where you want to go.

I will introduce you to some very powerful cash flow generating skill sets that you may have never considered—I've been doing this for a few years, all over the world, and I am being paid a lot of money for it.

I'll show you how and why your profits will never come from first time customers but from the sale after the sale.

*The Big Shift* was never meant to be a manual for everything you have to do to start and grow your flourishing business, because things change so fast. Tactics are short term. Strategic principles underpin your long-term business.

I'm going to break all that internet noise down into simple, easy-to-understand and do elements, and in my final chapter, I will ask you the most difficult question you'll need to answer—for yourself, and nobody else.

Who ever said that retirement is when you stop work, live on a golf course, and wait to die?  It's the working on what you love that ultimately leads to fulfillment, and buying back the lost years in corporate slavery.

So, let's get started on your journey.

I can't wait for you to race to the next chapter, where you'll discover that your start as an entrepreneur is NEVER about the product or idea you're going to create. It's about something that you know very personally, which is unique to you.

It's about you.

I'll be talking to you on the next page.

# Chapter 2

# Get Out of Your Head

*"It is easy to hate, and it is difficult to love. This is how the whole scheme of things works. All good things are difficult to achieve; and bad things are very easy to get."*
– Confucius

## Sacred Cows and Self-Limiting Beliefs

I've travelled the world and have spoken extensively to thousands of people looking to start a new business. But everyone that I've trained, including audiences of highly educated corporate types, academics, business owners, or just about anyone trying to start a business...regardless of who they are, they all share a single common theme that is keeping them where they are: stuck...in their own mind about money.

The money is the biggest thing you need to identify and fix before you start putting pen to paper, to go into business for yourself.

I was *that guy* too. I had a hard time. I don't want you to make that same mistake, so I'm sharing what took me a while to figure out.

Here's the fact...

You've been molded into false limiting beliefs about money; beliefs that you've been taught to hold true and steadfast. And you're not supposed to challenge it. But changing your false money concepts is going to be very critical on your way forward. And it starts with recognising what these money beliefs are.

Every time I list out the following to my business start-up entrepreneur clients (what Robert Kiyosaki refers to as the "Sacred Cows of Money"), there's always a smile and a laugh, because they've all heard it before...from their parents:

- Go to school
- Get a job
- Work hard
- Live below your means
- Save money
- Your house is an asset
- Get out of debt
- Diversify long-term investments

But there's always about ten percent of clients I teach that give me the best, most satisfying reaction of all: They sink into their seats with the look of pain, discomfort...and anger. These are the clients that are sick and tired of being sick and tired. They're ready to confront reality.

They're ready to make the big shift. And I know I can help them.

You already know that getting a college degree no longer guarantees lifetime employment. You may be qualified and skilled in a particular area of expertise, but college doesn't teach you how to make money. Joining the *rat race,* working 40 hours a week for the next 40 years, is also an old broken system. More and more jobs are on the line, and stress and depression weigh heavily on the shoulders of the employee as the company looks for different ways to cut costs and grow profits.

Living below your means is like telling yourself you don't deserve and are not worthy to enjoy the fruits of your labor. This philosophy on life destroys the spirit and soul, because you're telling yourself you're not good enough.

If you're leaving money in the bank, you're actually losing money with interest rates at zero, the devaluation of currency, and inflation. Your house is only an asset if it puts money in your pocket each month through net rental income, after management expenses, utilities, and mortgage interest payments.

Get out of debt? This is a good one. We've been taught that debt is bad. The financially educated know that there is good debt and bad debt. Good debt allows you to borrow money from a bank or from somebody else, or even from your credit card, to invest in things that ultimately make you money at a faster rate of return than the cost of borrowing. That's the chief reason why most adults don't continue to invest in their own education after college, as they think it costs them money without any return on value...plus they're already burdened with student loan debt.

You've likely invested in a mutual fund with a diversified portfolio, promising double-digit annual returns. What your manager isn't telling you, buried in the convoluted, overwhelming, fine-print legal language, are the monthly administration and management fees, which are taking out a chunk of your portfolio growth, which counters the positive effect of compound growth over the investing period. The people managing your fund are basically taking away a huge chunk of your future nest egg.

This may sound like *gibberish* to you—but it's not your fault—because you were never taught how money works, or how to generate cash flow with leverage, or how to make money work harder for you, or even the compounding effects on money. These are not new ideas but have been around for a long time.

If a lightbulb just switched on in your head, or you're starting to get a little uncomfortable, then great. What's in your mind—all that crap that has been accumulating since birth—is actually limiting your full potential. You need to start unlearning it, and you're not going to like it.

So let's get uncomfortable.

## Enlarge Your Comfort Zone

I'm scared of heights, but at least it's less now, compared to a few years ago. I'm sure there's a little vertigo in all of us. I mean, I can't be the only one who feels like being pulled to jump off a building when I'm peering over the edge, right?

They say F.E.A.R. is just an acronym for "False Emotions Appearing Real."

So, I decided to put this to the test.

One time, I was training an elite business clientele at a mastermind in Costa Rica, and during the course of the week-long program, we had a half-day off on day three to do some outdoor activities. Zip lining became my thing that day, when I decided to step into my fear.

We took a tractor trailer up the side of a mountain forest, about 500 feet above the forest floor. The course consisted of 15 zip lining stations and a narrow platform erected around the top of these gigantic tropical rain forest trees. My group passed the safety briefing, and one after another, we were pushed off the ledge as we flew across to the other tree, 300 feet off the ground. It was my turn. I let go and clung on for dear life. I absolutely screamed my head off as I flew through the jungle, the wind chilling every droplet of sweat on my skin from the fear I was experiencing. There was the deafening screeching sound of metal on metal as a pulley wheel above my head slid me down the steel line onto the next station platform.

The rush of adrenaline was unbelievable. I wanted more. And I completed the rest of the 14 stations in absolute exhilaration. I even have a souvenir picture of me hanging upside down, gazing at the forest floor below me.

I've been zip lining ever since, on every mastermind in Costa Rica that I've been hosting. Frankly, right now, it's getting boring. I've stared fear straight in the eye, smiled, and all of a sudden, I'm ready for the next challenge.

I just enlarged my comfort zone.

In my experience, the best way to grow is to constantly live on your edge of comfort, and push over just a little. Bit by bit, you become accustomed to a new level of self-awareness. All of a sudden, what was uncomfortable yesterday is your new comfort level today. As human beings, we have the greatest skill of adaptability. So, there is actually no such thing as a comfort zone. There is *lazy*, but not a comfort zone. To live life is to be challenged and stimulated. And we need to be constantly pushed outside our bubble.

I've been to a lot of self-transformation and self-development workshops, and I have spent tens of thousands of dollars on courses and online training programs just to get my head in the right place. The corporate world invested a lot in me: to be a better employee...for them. It's likely that they're also investing a lot in you right now. The problem is that your training and development has been biased to your performance in a set, clearly defined company operating structure.

You don't know it yet, but the day you leave that company, voluntarily or involuntarily, all that training will become useless (not all, but most of it for sure). You'll go from a predictable environment to the real world of business, where everything is but predictable.

You're going to be on your own.

As an entrepreneur, you need to learn a completely new set of skills just to make it. And that's going to require learning new things, doing different things, and thinking differently.

With anything new and important and worthwhile, you're going to get uncomfortable in the process.

The hard technical skills you acquired over your many years in your career are going to be important and transferable into your new business: third party business partners, developing systems and processes, accounting skills, professional qualifications, leading teams, product development, advertising, brand development, designing, customer service, sales, and so on. But as an entrepreneur, you need a completely different set of skills, many of which are not the hard skills that you have built up and stacked over years working for a company. It's the soft skills that require a high degree of emotional intelligence.

For example, you're a supervisor to your team in your current job, or a project leader, or a head of a department. You have assumed leadership by way of your title and company hierarchy. Your people don't really have a say in whether to follow you or not. On the other hand, as an entrepreneur, leadership is earned from the people who choose to follow you. That's when soft skills come in.

Another one is being a perfectionist. Stop it!! As an employee, we have to do a perfect job that is acceptable to our bosses. As a business owner, however, perfection is the enemy of progress. As long as things are stuck in your brain, or stuck in your computer, and it's not being put out into the marketplace, you're not making any money. Remember this: "Version 1.0 is infinitely better than 0.0" (quote from Brendon Burchard). Get your idea out there first, and make incremental improvements along the way.

I watched a YouTube video by a prominent consultant who said that most typical senior company executives actually fail at starting their own business. And I've known a few who didn't make it outside the corporate world. They can't get past their ego. There is so much wrapped around your name card, your office, and your car, as well as your reputation and social status in the community; and at work, you have a secretary, and a department you can command to run...all that goes away once you're out in the real world.

You're going to feel very lonely.

You need to find the big reason and the "why" behind your business. The reason why you're going to do the most courageous thing by becoming an entrepreneur with the tide against you, has to be big enough to overcome all that crap that's going to come your way. No one ever attempts the seemingly impossible without the belief in something or someone greater than themselves.

It's going to be critically important that the seed of your business idea that's in your brain gets protected, nurtured, incubated, and looked after. It must be nourished, sown, reaped, and harvested in the fertile environment you create and allow into your new life.

## The Average of 5: Broke or Billionaire?

The great Jim Rohn once said, in one of his many famous quotes, *"You are the average of the five people you spend the most time with."* This is one of the most frequently quoted and inspiring quotes that successful people refer to, because it's true.

I remember the first time that I hung out with a multi-millionaire online business entrepreneur in Thailand. He told me the story of growing up in a neighbourhood of shady characters, drug dealers, and gangsters. "That environment only gives you two choices", he said. "Become a drug dealer or get killed in the process." So, when he chose to do something completely different from the people around him, he told me he took out his phone and started deleting every single contact in his address book that he knew would drag him back down into the gutter.

Here's a short exercise for you—just humor me for a bit.

Take out a piece of paper and write down the names of the five people you spend the most time with in a given week. But you can't include immediate family members; you can't delete them from your life. Note: All other relatives are fair game.

For each person, write down what they do for a living, and take an educated guess at how much they make in a year. Add up all those salaries and divide it by five, which will give you an average for your group.

I'll bet you that you're earning within 15 to 20 percent of that average. Now, imagine what each of them would say if you told them that you're quitting your job to start your own business.

What do you think each of them would say to you, or even what their reaction and look on their face would be?

I've traveled the world extensively as an international speaker and trainer, and I've had the privilege of meeting a lot of amazing people, including people with extraordinary stories that I've shared the stage with. I remember meeting one guy who is an absolute expert in e-commerce, making hundreds of thousands of dollars in sales across multiple niches. He was also an adrenaline junkie.

He worked as a deep sea crab fisherman, off the coast of Alaska, for five years. And this was out of choice. Have you ever watched these crazy fishing programs on the Discovery Channel, where these guys are overshadowed by hundred-foot waves, working on a trawler in atrocious conditions, in freezing rain storms? Well, this guy was one of them.

After hauling in a major catch, he would have to dump the crabs into huge, deep buckets, and would watch them. Just for fun, he would dangle a rope down into the bucket and watch a crab hold onto it and try to climb out. But what was amazing to watch was that all the other crabs, piled on top of each other inside that bucket, would reach up with their claws and pull the escaping crab back into the bucket.

That story illustrates the challenge of the entrepreneur against the environment they're in. Not only will other people who don't believe in you pull you down, you too can drag yourself back into the bucket just by sabotaging your own dreams.

That image is so powerful, and it'll stick with me for life.

## The Power of a Mentor and a Coach

I've been regularly speaking and training in 4 continents, and I always get asked by my clients and students about the keys to success: "What's the *one single thing* that made the biggest difference in your journey?"

Everyone asks me that because most people starting a new business are looking for that one quick fix, that one shortcut to riches. Amateurs look for that lottery ticket. Newsflash guys: It's a grind; the professional knows and accepts it. However, there are ways to compress that time and shorten the learning curve.

It has always been down to a mentor and a coach, and they're two very different things. The biggest leaps forward on my journey were made by having both at the same time, in short bursts, to help me overcome a specific challenge or blockage.

A coach has a vested interest in your results. That's why coaches get fired when the athlete isn't winning. A coach will help you maximize your skills and talents toward a result, and if they can't, another coach will replace them and try to do the same.

A mentor, on the other hand, has minimal stake in your end results. Whether or not you succeed makes no difference to them. It's a harsh way of putting it, but it's true. Of course, they will celebrate your success, while preserving themselves in the face of any hurdles or failures you face along the way. A mentor takes a longer-term view of where you're heading; they will tell you next level advice or guide you on what next strategic element you'll need to consider, and make it make sense for your business.

For example, one of my mentors gave me just one piece of advice that literally changed the way I marketed my business: copywriting. Find the top books written on the topic, and learn copywriting. That was it!! So, that's what I did. I bought ten books, read them all, and started implementing. In the space of just a couple of months, I was converting leads with my landing pages and funnels, at over 35%, and along with a joint venture partner, we did six-figures in under 6 months.

My mentor never taught me how to implement. He gave me a *flick on the ear*, telling me to scrap this, junk that, and learn this.

If you're lucky enough to be surrounded or have access to good people who believe in you and can offer sound coaching or mentoring advice, then great. The majority of the time, coaches and mentors charge a fee because they know their advice can potentially change the course of your business, and help you launch your product in the millions of dollars; or they can take a business to a completely new level that you never even thought of. So, you need to set aside a budget and go look for a coach and a mentor—ideally, both.

The kind of mentor or coach that you want to choose is someone who has the kind of lifestyle that you're looking for—someone who has the success that you're aiming for, who shares your values, and is not afraid to tell you what you need to know, and not what you want to hear.

Over the years, I've invested over $150,000 in paid coaching and mentoring on my business journey. People around me thought I was absolutely crazy. But what they didn't understand— and it took me a long time to change my thinking and approach to money and investing in myself in this way—was that I knew if I could take one insight from their experience that could save me 6 months and avoid a lot more money trying to figure it out on my own, then it would be worth it. If that investment could translate into at least achieving that level of revenue increase and more, that would be a great return on my investment.

But there's another secret, a hidden value and benefit of investing in the right kind of mentor. And it happened to me 12 months after I hired my first one.

They open doors for you.

The only reason I got into speaking (we'll cover platform speaking later in the book) was because a mentor I invested in opened doors for me. Beyond the advice for your own development and how to run your business, they also bring you access to a greater network of possibilities, opportunities, and individuals.

And that's the real value you're getting.

## Burn the Boats

The expression, *burn the boats*, traces back to the Spanish conquest of Mexico, by commander Hernan Cortes, who destroyed his ships so that his men would either conquer or die. It means to continue one's course of action because turning back is too dangerous, physically impossible, too expensive, or too painful.

I *burned my boats* years ago when I found out that going back to a job was not an option. I could no longer handle the commute; neither could I navigate around internal politics, nor the pride-swallowing siege of not being paid my worth, and handing over my time to someone else, knowing that one day, I would be at their mercy of either maintaining the livelihood for my family, or being made redundant again.

I was never going to let my life be in someone else's hands again.

Most of today's job mentality is to not do too much and avoid the extra stress, or doing just enough not to get fired. The traditional workplace is a terrible environment to realise your full potential. And as organisations become flatter, the climb up the ladder has become even more competitive for the fewer and fewer jobs that are above you.

There are two types of employees these days: *hiders* and *movers*. The *hiders* are those who put in the minimum necessary just to get by. They don't voice their opinions out of fear, and are typically passing the buck. *Movers* stand out and end up doing everything possible to climb that ladder, except doing their job.

There are those, within each of the two types, who have the entrepreneurial spirit inside them, whether they realise it or not. They have lost motivation at work because they're looking for more; or they are the overachievers who can't get what they truly want, and end up leaving to build their own ventures. But they remain in their jobs just long enough so that they can understand how an organisation functions, and how a business works, and plan to prepare themselves for the biggest shift in their life, in becoming an entrepreneur.

They are crafting their business plan while still in their job.

But you need to *burn your boats* if you're ever going to make it as an entrepreneur. You have to have the inner conviction, a fire burning in your soul, that you're going to do whatever it takes, that you're all in, there is no Plan B, and that everything you do from this point forward is going to focus your entire energy and your entire being, into you, into your success, into your family, and into whatever purpose you set out to achieve.

Here are a few practical tips that I give clients when they start their journey as a business owner with the expertise they already have, even while they're still in a job.

When you understand these tips, they will begin to encapsulate the kind of disciplined mindset and habits that you have to start adopting as an entrepreneur. The good news is that you're already doing them in your job. The bad news is that you need to do them while no one's watching.

So, here are 10 entrepreneurial productive habits to get you started:

1.  Devote one hour a day on feeding your mind, ideally in the morning.

2.  Combine this with writing down and reciting your gratitude and what you want to achieve in life, and how that feels. It is best to do this first thing in the morning when you wake up, or sing it while taking your morning shower—a personal favorite of mine!

3.  Decide how many hours a week you will devote to starting your business. You decide whether the week is Monday to Friday, to Sunday, or just certain days and times in the week. But stick to it by scheduling it as a meeting in your diary; set an alarm and reminder, and make sure you show up on time.

4.  Set your mobile to timer mode, and give yourself the allotted time to accomplish what you need to accomplish. Switch off all email and social media notifications, and get to work. By having a visual timer next to you, you imprint in your brain to work toward a deadline. Whether it's designing a product or service, a product map, a branding strategy, a lead-

generation plan, or a customer acquisition funnel, this is an incredibly productive session, and you'll be blown away at how productive you can be as you begin building the pieces of the puzzle to your new business. I usually set work tasks for one hour and no more. Then, move on to the next.

5.  Give yourself a specific work objective for that time allocation. Don't leave it to creative inspiration, because your mind will wander into social media land...and nothing will get done. Say to yourself, "In 1 hour, I will complete and finish XYZ task." It could be outlining or writing a business plan, designing a product value ladder, or making phone calls to leads or potential partners and investors—whatever that is, make it specific and achievable in your work time. A business takes form as a result of the sum of the individual small parts. Question: "How do you eat a 10-ton elephant?" Answer: "One piece at a time." I think you get it now!

6.  Focus on these three areas in your dedicated time, and eliminate anything that doesn't fall into these buckets: Create, Communicate, Convert. Creating a product or service for selling is one of the most productive, money-making activities you can do that will translate into profits down the road. Start communicating now what you will be selling and marketing 6 months from now; create anticipation in the marketplace. You can do this by conducting online surveys to better understand your audience, or start doing branded posts to build curiosity (I'll cover this in the next chapter.). Converting is making sales. You may not be ready yet, but a step before a paying customer, is generating leads of prospects, or even anyone who is interested in what you have to say. Building a database of leads now, will translate into paying customers later, when your product is released.

7.  If distractions at home are an issue, I found that my own most productive environment, ironically, is actually in a cafe. Grab your favourite beverage, put on your favourite tunes, make sure you get your hands on a good set of noise-cancelling headphones, and get to work. The only distraction you will have will be when you have to go to the bathroom...nothing else.

8.  One of my earliest working environments was investing in a monthly membership to a co-work space (Okay, I didn't have a job to go to, so I created the habit of going to an office for the day.). The space had great interior decor, and I was surrounded by start-up folks, and it actually felt like work. This is just a suggestion, if that's the habit ramp you need to be on to trigger you into productivity *beast mode*. Plus, it allows you to network with others. Believe me, the vibe is different, and others are genuinely interested in what you're working on.

9.  Subscribe to top marketer websites and other industries you particularly like, or are related to your business area; then analyze and take screenshots of every step you are navigating through, from welcome emails and newsletters, to how their links are set-up, to selling propositions, to their use of copy. Buy from websites to see how these companies deliver, fulfill, and follow through with customer support. This goes to building up a picture of how that company or expert markets online through *funnels*. (Don't worry; we're going to cover that later in the book too!)

10. Find groups or networking events around the industry where you have a business to market into. Use that opportunity to fine-tune your product or service idea from networking with people in this industry. Chances are, you probably know your target audience problem, and you're

using these networking opportunities to fine-tune your product idea.

If you're used to working against a task list in your job, then this shouldn't be a big deal. The biggest challenge will be to be disciplined on it, because you're the only one accountable to yourself. And that's why your mindset and motivation is so important.

I can't wait for you to rush into the next chapter, where I'm going to reveal, explain, and teach you one of the most important things about you and your business, which you need to create so that you can begin attracting future customers, by sheer presence of what you stand for, becoming the hunted and not the hunter.

# Chapter 3

# YOU, Inc.

*"The higher your energy level, the more efficient your body. The more efficient your body, the better you feel and the more you will use your talent to produce outstanding results."*
– Tony Robbins

## The Land of Me-Too

So, you've got a business idea. You have a pretty good idea of what your target audience is looking for, and how you're going to solve their problems with your innovative, revolutionary idea that's going to be the best thing since sliced bread.

But that's the easy part. The next, and likely most challenging, part to any new business is how you are going to find customers and generate that much needed cash-flow.

Your customers are individuals who started out as leads or prospects. These are people who saw your ad and raised their hand in curiosity to want to find out more. That is simply a lead. Now, imagine this: What if instead of chasing after leads by bombarding them with expensive advertising, or by getting referrals from your friends, and ending up only turning them off to what you have to say about your product...what if leads and prospects flowed effortlessly into your business, like crazy shoppers rushing into your store because of who you are in their mind's eye?

What if your customers hunted you down, instead of you hunting them?

Imagine these crazy fans of your product, who only chose YOU each and every time, and not anybody else who arguably has a similar product or service that could equally deliver a solution with similar results to what you have to offer?

What makes you special?   And how do you differentiate yourself from everybody else in the *land of me-too*?

Branding.

I'm going to let you in on a little secret: the truth behind branding. It's not a real secret because, intuitively, you as a consumer, as a shopper, already know this. So, I'm just going to help you reconnect the dots, and illuminate a new perspective to you on branding.

I worked my whole life in marketing and sales, and I've been schooled by one of the most reputable companies that, back in the day, was widely recognised as the real world business school of marketing. When I started my career, there were only a handful of companies that were renowned for their approach to branding: Procter and Gamble, Johnson and Johnson, Unilever, Coca-Cola, and Philip Morris.

They were the real business schools of marketing.

I worked at Philip Morris for close to 18 years, as a senior executive on many of their famous brands, and nothing is more recognizable than the brand, *Marlboro*. In the mid-1990s, Marlboro was consistently among the top 10 most valuable brands in the world, according to global brand consultancy firm, Interbrand. I still have an old clipping from 1995, when Coca-Cola just edged out Marlboro in becoming the most valuable brand in the world. In a December, 1996 *New York Times* article, Marlboro was referred to alongside several other mega brands that made the top 10 list that year, including McDonald's; the Walt Disney Company; Kodak, from the Eastman Kodak Company; Sony; Gillette; Mercedes-Benz, sold by Daimler-Benz A.G.; Levi's; and Microsoft.

So, putting all the controversy and bad stuff aside about big tobacco, I know something about branding.

What comes to your mind when I mention the brand, Coca-Cola? Red? Happy? Children? A jolly Santa Claus? By the way, there is a conspiracy theory in marketing circles that *Santa Claus* was a character invented by Coca-Cola, as a commercial marketing ploy to sell more Coke.

What about McDonald's? Ronald McDonald?

How about when I say *Apple*? Great design? White? Raving fans? Three-mile long line into an Apple store, ahead of the launch of a new iPhone? Or perhaps the face of Steve Jobs?

What comes to your mind when I mention these major brands?

Now, I use these brand examples to illustrate a point, but you take any brand that you can think of, including accounting firms, law firms, banks, or any other company that manufactures a product or is behind a service. It doesn't have to be on a supermarket shelf.

A brand is not just a logo. It's not made up from a dizzying array of business metrics, valuations, market capitalization, and formulas. A brand is a personification of an idea. We buy brands because we buy people who relate to us as individuals, as human beings. We buy brands because, deep down inside, we're buying into trust.

It's the same in today's digital world as it has always been.

A brand is actually a person.

## Why Brand Yourself?

We think brands only relate to everyday consumer products we find in our local grocery store, supermarket, or even on Amazon. Not true. Regardless of the product or service behind your business idea, the only way you can win customers is if you can get your brand personality to become an extension of who you are and what you stand for, so that when customers buy your brand, they're actually buying YOU.

You are unique. Therefore, your brand, by definition, is unique and different from the sea of sameness.

So, why do you need to brand yourself or your business? There are too many other people and other businesses trying to market and sell the same thing as you, and you're not going to stand out unless you have a brand.

Let's face it; we live in an ADHD society—we have the attention span of a fish. People buy from people. In this information overloaded world and commercial noise, we've become cynical and numb. It takes a lot to excite us these days. Yet the world suddenly wakes up to cat videos, with a global resonating,

"Ahhhhh!!!" We're looking for empathy in a faceless, cold, cut-throat world of pain. We're looking to connect with another human being...on a human level.

A brand gives you a competitive edge so that you can charge more in a competitive marketplace, your product performs better, or you have stratospheric customer service in the way you support your customers. Your product should never appeal on price alone. Pricing is an unprofitable business strategy because it means you are prepared to undercut your competition and drain your profits. Nobody benefits with pricing, as it drags the industry down into a never-ending spiral.

Branding is what keeps companies profitable and efficient.

You might be thinking that branding is only for big companies and everyday consumer products that people buy in stores. You may have a consulting business. You may want to start a real-estate business. You're into gardening. You're into building and construction. Every idea needs a brand behind it in order for it to be sellable and to stand out from every other similar idea.

All you need now is to make a shift away from your misinformed perception about branding.

Branding is about building an attractive character to your audience.

## Finding Your Inner Attractive Character

So, let's get down to the *nitty gritty* of figuring out your brand. Remember, a brand is a person; a personification that embodies everything of who you are. So, why do we like the people we like in our lives? Why do we dislike some people and are unsure about others?

We tend to like other people like us. Or we like other people who are the kind of people we want to become.

It comes down to character. And it starts with a major problem.

Virgin Atlantic is an airline company that was started by Sir Richard Branson, who created the Virgin brand of companies. That airline was born out of frustration, and a problem. When Branson bought and started building his paradise getaway at Necker Island, there weren't any direct flights from London to the British Virgin Islands. So, he created Virgin Atlantic, battled and won the biggest lawsuit in the industry against British Airways. Blinkist, an app with over 10 million users that lets you read the key lessons from over 3,000 non-fiction books, was started by a group of guys working in jobs who wanted to continue to read and learn but didn't have the time. Shopify, the world's leading e-commerce platform, was started in Canada by Tobias Lutke, Daniel Weinand, and Scott Lake, who wanted to sell snowboard gear online, but there just wasn't any good software at the time to do the job the way they wanted it done.

Big brands are created by founders, out of a profound problem that they were passionate to solve for themselves; and they made a fortune by solving similar problems for millions of other people around the world.

Notice in these examples how each entrepreneur had a backstory behind solving the problem they faced. It doesn't matter if it's a physical product or service; your business idea that you feel passionate about stems from a problem that you're facing. The fortune is this: There are millions of other people around the world with that same problem. You just need to solve it for them, better than anyone else.

So, you need to craft your attractive character, which contains a backstory, so that people can resonate with your dilemma, and they will want to know how *you're* able to solve that same problem *they're* facing today.

The key elements of crafting your attractive character includes a backstory with lots of emotions and frustrations, parables and lessons learnt, and how you came up with a better way of doing things.

The network marketing industry thrives on stories of individuals who went from *rags to riches*. The skin care and weight loss industry uses a story angle of a *before-and-after* punchline. The better the human emotion, the more resonating the story.

We love to root for the underdog. We are inspired by victory overcoming defeat. We are touched by good conquering evil. This is the classic story blueprint for the majority of Hollywood movies today.

One of the best and most powerful ways you can win over your leads and prospects is when you identify the *common enemy*: the government, healthcare, taxes, education, drug companies, the food industry, big corporate, fraud, scammy travel agency websites, and expensive hotels. Many brands and industries have emerged, and have won millions of fans as a result of the common enemy: Airbnb, alternative medicine, the organic food industry, CBD oils.

We are in the opportunity of the alternative niche. Decades ago, it was about big business. If you wanted to start a business, you needed to cater to the masses. Today, there is an over-proliferation of mass commercial products, and consumer preferences have changed to more authentic alternative choices.

Just look at the resurgence of brands like Puma, Adidas Classics (the three-leaf clover logo), and New Balance, and now a mass of very niche alternative brands that challenge the big corporate brand houses.

The back-to-retro trend is the result of people going back to what works, nostalgia, and most importantly, trust.

This is the reason why people gravitate toward new, highly targeted brands that have an individual and personal flare.

Big corporate is being threatened by small start-ups and home-based entrepreneurs.

And that sets the stage for you.

## The 4 Archetypes

Once you have your back story, you now need to frame it around 4 key character types: *Charger, Experiencer, Journalist,* and *Silent Giver.*

*Chargers* sit on the cutting edge of innovation. They've discovered a new way of doing things. They are creating a revolution. They're creating a paradigm shift within a specific niche of an industry. If you are a Charger, you typically position yourself as a leading expert that challenges the status quo, and that shifts beliefs and mindsets and perceptions into moving toward a better solution.

An *Experiencer* is one who shares personal experiences and testimonials about using a particular product or service. Hence, companies today pay a lot of money for social media influencers to endorse their product or perform a demo on camera—even a video just on unwrapping the packaging! Foodies are also a great example of an Experiencer. They take pictures of the foods they explore; they travel the world and allow us to experience vicariously the multitude of cuisines and delicacies from all over the world.

The *Journalist* uses third party experiences, expertise, and testimonials to provide different perspectives on a given topic. If you are the Journalist character, you are seen as an expert, not necessarily because you are the go-to person on the subject matter, but because you bring expert content and resources that tap into a network of knowledge and credible authorities to convey insights to the viewer.

And finally, a *Silent Giver* is the type of person who secretly discovered a solution, a shortcut, or an innovative piece of software that drastically solves a huge problem. This person is not looking for fame or fortune but now has a selfless greater responsibility to the world to share it.

You can now see that each of these four character types are equally attractive in their own way. The subtle differences between them is how they convey their information through their persona to the world. The *Charger* and the *Experiencer* typically PUSH their discoveries out to the world; the *Journalist* and the *Silent Giver* PULL the viewer into their world.

This is a crucial step before you start formulating and structuring your brand and how it will represent you out in the world.

Defining your brand is a painful journey and does take time because of the distillation process of compressing everything you want to try to do, right down into its core DNA.

What is your brand ultimately about?

When I train clients on this process, it may take hours for some, if not weeks for others. There is a lot of soul searching. There is frustration. I've gone through weeks when my clients weren't responding because I challenged their thinking process. However, once you commit yourself to the process of soul-searching, and you remain open and disciplined, you and your brand will become a magnet to a world of consumers who need and will pay for your product, over and over again.

Once you crack your attractive character, the next part of the process of defining your brand becomes a lot smoother.

## The BrandQ Methodology™

I developed The BrandQ Methodology™ some years ago; although, admittedly, I didn't have a name for it back then. I started teaching this approach to branding your business to my mastermind clients, because they knew the importance of branding, yet they were so confused by all the complicated theories and jargon that were out there.

Big companies have made a complete science behind designing a brand, and for the novice, you need a PhD in astrophysics to be able to decipher the intricacies and sheer mental popcorn and teeth-pulling that exists in the agency and branding world in creating these icons. But these approaches have been mastered from decades of evolution, and billions of dollars of investment, which explains why we're witnessing some of the most valuable brands in the world that have captured our hearts.

As a start-up entrepreneur, you can't take the same process that has built billion dollar brands, and apply it to your own startup idea, nor do you need to. So that's why I fine-tuned The BrandQ Methodology into something simple and intellectually painless, so that you can start bringing mega brand thinking into your start-up business.

The BrandQ Methodology centers on "You Incorporated," or simply, "You Inc.," because the brand is built around YOU. And YOU are your ultimate asset.

Here's a sketch of what that looks like:

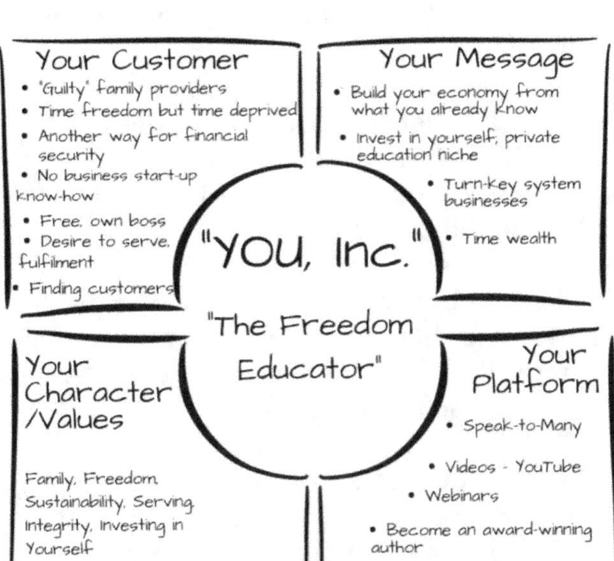


Print-ready, downloadable worksheet available at www.MakeTheBigShiftBook.com

My methodology comprises 4 quadrants (hence, the Q), with "YOU Inc.," your brand, bang in the middle.

For illustration, I've completed this by replicating a picture of my own brand to show you how the methodology works.

The top left quadrant is about your ideal customer or client. It's about the single biggest problem they're facing, their hopes and dreams, and their biggest pain and fears. This is less about your target demographic like age, income, etc. It's the insight of what drives them forward and what holds them back. The shorter the phrase, the clearer the picture of your ideal customer.

Take my ideal client as an example: Working parents provide for the family but feel guilty for missing out on their children growing up. They want time freedom but are time deprived. They're looking for a better way to have more time, while securing a financial safety net. They have a desire to serve. They want the freedom of being their own boss but don't know how to start a business. Or they have already started a business but are struggling to find customers.

The bottom left quadrant is about your character values that you uphold as true, and that also resonates and is relevant to your ideal customer. For me, it's family, freedom, sustainability, serving, integrity, and self-investment.

The top right is your message to the world: your key talking points if you were to sit down in a cafe with your ideal customer sitting right in front of you. Another perspective is what advice you would give yourself, knowing what you know now. These are the things I would say to my ideal client: "Build income-producing assets on what you already know. The opportunity is in commercialized education and investing in yourself. Turn-key systems are the key to future-proofing your business.

Become time-wealthy; everything you do must free up time for you, as it is the most precious asset you have."

And finally, the 4th quadrant is about the platform and method that best gets your message out to the world. It is the perfect medium and megaphone that works best for you. If your ideas are best conveyed through words, then write a book, or journal or blog. If you are a conversationalist, learn how to speak to many. Get in front of a camera and film video blogs, start a podcast, or do all three.

Once you figure out this final quadrant that best magnifies who you are, what your message is, and how your customers will find you, you will then be crystal clear on what you want to achieve with social media, and avoid wasted time, and focus on trying to do everything.

In my business, my brand messages are best conveyed through speaking from the big stage, videos, and webinars, and being an award-winning author. Those aren't the only platforms I use in marketing my message, but they are the ones that I enjoy doing, and where I feel my message comes through in the best possible way.

And that's it! The BrandQ Methodology. I told you it was simple.

If you'd like to download a high quality, print-ready version of The BrandQ Methodology diagram, for you to complete yourself, or even with me over a free consultation call, just head over to my website, at www.MakeTheBigShiftBook.com, for this free bonus and more that comes with this book.

If you'd like some help working through it, just drop me a message at the same website.

In the next chapter, you're going to find out how to get your message out there and never run out of ideas to talk about. You'll also learn about the one thing that will be your biggest salesman, who will be working for you around the clock, 24 hours a day, 7 days a week, 365 days a year, and will never ask for vacation.

I can't wait to show you what's coming around the corner...

# Chapter 4

# Your Megaphone

*"Most people say that it is the intellect which makes a great scientist.*
*They are wrong: it is character."*
– Albert Einstein

## Who's Listening?

Here are 6 key truths, and your *modus operandi,* as you begin crafting and implementing the strategy behind your marketing messages:

- Your customers and clients buy into your story...and will buy from you.

- Your stories are memorable.

- Give them a nugget of insight at every point of contact.

- Address their pain...and convey the benefits of your solution.

- Variety keeps you interesting.

- And most of all, your customers and clients want to BELIEVE.

The biggest fear that my coaching clients have in getting their message out to the world is the fear that whatever they have to say will be ridiculed, or that it's not good enough.

I don't buy their insecurity. They've lived and worked for so many years, and to think they have nothing to say is actually a fear that will keep them where they are in life. It's selfish not to share your insights to the world, especially when your knowledge can help tens of thousands of people with their problems. The beauty of this is, you can profit from it with integrity, because you will have helped somebody progress out of their situation.

Someone once told me, "Move from being a consumer of content...to a producer of content."

That's a success mindset.

In this world, there are three types of people, and a direct correlation to the income leverage they can generate.

There are people who DO, without much thinking. These are typically employees who trade their time for a paycheck.

The second type of person DOES BETTER with some level of THINKING. They are typically self-employed people who have a business but are still trading an hourly rate for money. They do better than a salaried employee, but they still don't have much leverage, because they can't create more hours in a day to charge clients...unless they give up sleep!

The third type sells HOW TO DO THINGS BETTER. In other words, they sell thinking.

These individuals typically have built a system that sells products and services that teaches people around the world how to be more effective and efficient.

I'll be teaching you, later in the book, how to start to create your own products and services with a system that can leverage your time and make you a lot of money with stuff you already know.

## Strive to Be the Better Teacher with Endless Content

My biggest mentoring advice to you is this: Strive to become the best teacher and educator in your niche. Don't aim for the perfect product or the perfect service or the perfect system. Your goal is to be the better teacher than anyone else out there.

What you know and have learnt from experience in all your years in the workplace, is invaluable, and can't be found in traditional academic establishments. HINT: You can take a pretty good guess at how much Harvard University charges for a *useless* MBA degree these days. They're in the business of selling their brand and credibility...and are doing this using outdated business cases!

Let's talk about where you can find content to teach others in your chosen platform, through writing, filming, or recording an audio about it. Here are my 4 keys to never be struggling to find marketing content to talk about in your messaging:

#1: **Teach what you're reading.** You'll be amazed to know that just by reading 3 books on a given topic, automatically qualifies you as an expert.

One of the biggest sources of my content for educating people on financial education, entrepreneur startup, and marketing was through reading books. I created a library of over 160 videos on my YouTube channel, and all I did, after each chapter of a book, was to write  3 key takeaways, and then convert it into a short, 4-minute video blog. (I'll reveal my *4-Steps to 4-Minute Videos Formula,* in a later chapter.)

**#2:  Transpose what you watch and learn, into a content piece.** There is just so much video content out on the internet, and there is nothing you can't learn that isn't already on YouTube. The secret is that you don't have to originate your own breakthrough idea content; you can just provide your own perspective on what you learned, and it automatically becomes an original piece. Same idea: Convert that learning into 1, 2, or 3 bullet points, write a blog around it, and record a video or audio.

**#3:  Express empathy with something, and how it inspired you to talk about it.** This way just adds a little bit of variety in your content, which shows that you're human. Get used to witnessing stories and turning them around into a lesson that teaches the viewer or reader something about what you're an expert in. Yes, you have to teach what you're an expert in, but you can't be a one-trick pony all the time. This is about rounding out your overall brand character by introducing variety in your content.

Remember our flooded apartment?  I recorded a YouTube video, a couple days later, on the experience, with the message of asset protection.

**#4: Record the miracles that happen daily in your life.** People are hungry for hope, and are inspired by other people's stories. Teach people gratitude.

The way in which your brand attracts more interest than your competition is the better way behind how you teach it, and is less on what you're teaching. So learn to be the better teacher.

In summary, here's what to take away with you on building your branded content:

- Choose the best megaphone for your message that can reach the greatest number of people in the fastest way.

- You have to love creating content.

- Make it a habit.

- Invest in your craft.

- Be consistent.

## Everybody Needs a Funnel

I go through spurts of doing the right things to get back in shape. I go through months not following a healthy diet, but then I follow that up with 6 months of stuff to try to get me *shredded* (actually I've never managed to achieve this...but it's the intention that counts right?)...and then I fall back into my old reality again.

One day, while I was checking out fitness videos on YouTube, these annoying ads kept popping up. Some guy named Mike Chang was showing off his abs and literally getting in my face by telling me about the *one thing* why men over 40 will never look like he does...but finally can. This kept going on for days (you know how Google creeps up on you as soon as you click on something, and then all of a sudden, you are bombarded by the same stuff, over and over again!!). My world was suddenly inundated by Mike Chang!  He was this annoying voice in my head, and his videos were following me everywhere I browsed on the internet.

So I decided to watch the full length video ad. At the end, Mike told me to click on a link, which I did, because I now desperately wanted to watch that 26-minute video, where he promised to reveal what that *one thing* was. I entered my name and email address, got hold of that video—and it just blew me away.

I watched his story about growing up as a fat Asian kid, and then the video went into a scientific study and explanation about something to do with testosterone levels and leptin that gave men the *fanny pack* around their waistline.

I was sold once the pitch on Mike's supplements came on. I pulled out my credit card and bought a $300 kit of starter supplements, plus an exercise app of intense, short training exercises to burn fat. I even had these sleep tablets that contained melatonin that would burn fat while you slept—*riiiiiiight*!!

I used the exercise app for about 6 weeks and was really starting to feel good. I then got a call out of the blue from Cindy. I could just picture her in my mind: a blonde, sun-tanned, California babe. She greeted me with, *"Hey Ian, it's Cindy, from California. How're you doin' today?"* (head bob :))

"Good," I replied. "Except..." (as I look down at my belly), "...nothing's happening!"

She was my personal fitness consultant, and offered a special deal..."just for me." Needless to say, I pulled out my credit card AGAIN, and bought a couple more boxes of the stuff. They've been sitting on my kitchen shelf for 2 years and are going mouldy.

Guests would come over, see all those jars of tablets on the shelf, and say, with an impressive look on their face, "Wow, you're sure into your *SHELF-development!*"

The point of the story is that Mike Chang *sucked* me into his funnel and got me to buy—not once but twice. He was amazing; I loved his story, and I respect him for his new ventures in changing the lives of teens all across America today. Would I buy from him ever again? Of course I will. It's about his brand, and his attractive character.

Everyone needs a funnel. You do too.

A funnel is simply a step-by-step process that converts curiosity into cash.

In the old days (now I'm really giving up my age), we watched television, listened to the radio, read magazines, and saw billboards. Then we would go to the store and buy what we saw. That was a funnel, and we're always in somebody's funnel because we're always shopping. Something triggers our interest, which often leads us to make a purchase. Cha-Ching!!

With advancements in technology and social media platforms, companies and businesses are using very sophisticated means and funnels to *fish* for leads and customers.

I want to keep this complex topic simple, so focus on these basic principles and strategies, because every business, including your new start-up, must have a funnel...or several of them:

Every business needs new and repeat customers to start and grow.

A prospective customer starts as a lead, a person who raises their hand to take a look at your solution to the problem.

The role of advertising is to qualify leads, separating those who raise their hands after seeing the ad, from those who just saw the ad and will likely not buy from you...at least for now.

Your funnel is the process to convert those leads into pulling out their credit cards and becoming your buyers.

How well you convert leads depends on your funnel strategy.

How you ask people to buy at each funnel stage, and how much they pay you, determines how much money you make.

What's important when I train clients is for them to understand the principles and the strategy. Once they have this locked in, they can then go ahead and brief somebody else to help them build a funnel.

Normally, what I do with clients is walk through the process, where they come out with a clear blueprint and strategy for acquiring customers for their business. Then, with this blueprint, they simply have to hand it over to a digital marketer, who will do the funnel build-out for them.

For certain businesses that I have a particular affinity for, I actually project manage and build out their business funnels for them.

## The Long End of the Stick

Now, you've probably come across the saying, *"...getting the short end of the stick."* It's an expression for any customer who got a raw deal: an unfair, lop-sided arrangement that favored the seller more than the buyer.

In today's world, you have to have the psychology of giving your customer *"the long end of the stick."* What this simply means is to over-deliver, and give them more value than they paid for, and they will become lifelong, loyal customers of you and your business.

This is how it breaks down into execution...

I've spoken about creating funnels to generate leads and prospects. Unless you have a steady flow of leads, you don't have a prayer of getting a customer, because not everyone who sees your ad will buy. Leads are people who are interested and curious about what you have to offer through your business solution or product. They have the potential of becoming your customers, depending on how you nurture these leads over time and convert them.

Take, for instance, the Mike Chang funnel from a video ad he posted on YouTube. He lured me into clicking on a link, then baited me with a 26-minute video of value I wanted to learn about, and in exchange, I gave him my name and email address and became his lead. I then got an email link to some bonuses, and on the back of those, I ended up pulling out my credit card for my first purchase.

But the funnel didn't stop there...

I got on a *coaching* call with Cindy, who sold me more of the stuff, for a "special deal just for me!"

Because a lead read something about you, or they read something you wrote on a blog, or they watched a video of you teaching something that tweaked their curiosity, the likelihood of them giving you their name and email address increases by 10 times, because you have branded yourself in their eyes. You have become a credible authority and, hopefully, they are starting to trust you.

I had a level of trust with Mike Chang, having seen his ad a few times.

A lead magnet is something that is educational, insightful, or useful, and is related to what you were writing about, or what your video was about that got them interested, which you give away for free, in exchange for somebody's name and email address. Mike Chang's lead magnet was the 26-minute video on *the one thing* that was preventing men, over 40, from getting a visible 6-pack.

The beauty of digital marketing today is that we don't need physical inventory of the stuff we give away for free. A lot of these lead magnets today can be created in digital form and downloadable, simply by sending an automatic email as soon as someone opts in with their email address, and telling them to click on a link to download.

Here are some great tips for lead magnets: lists of secrets, hacks, short cuts, how-to's, fast ways, guaranteed results—things of that nature are typically very, very valuable, and what people want.

If you're in the real estate niche, perhaps it is: "Seven proven, bullet-proof ways to finding distressed home sellers and making you a fortune in less than 30 days." What frustrated realtor, who hasn't had a deal in months, wouldn't want a quick way to start earning cash?

Or, if you're in the accounting niche: "Six hidden loopholes to pay less taxes...legally."

How about if you're in the network marketing niche: "Here are the top 10 mistakes every average network marketer falls into, winding up never getting their business off the ground."

Focus on creating a lead magnet that addresses the biggest problem your target audience is facing.

So, you get what I'm talking about. Now, that's just the first stage of giving the "long end of the stick" to a potential lead or prospect.

The psychology of selling your business idea, product, or service is, whenever somebody chooses to follow you, or someone decides to give you their name and email address, you always want to over-deliver. When you sell your first product, always bundle it with bonuses. Bonus offers should either be complementary to the product they bought (e.g., get a case with a 24-pack set of pencils), or make the product they bought work even better (e.g., download *The Big Shift* MP3 audio version, and listen on-the-go—actually, this is a real, free bonus offer of several that I give away with this book. Just head to www.MakeTheBigShiftBook.com, and download yours right now.).

## Offer Them a Red Ferrari

Bonuses are a great way to win customers for life.

The following is true...

Dubai is a haven for the super-rich: a property market for the elite home buyers who have a few million bucks to splurge on an *out-of-this-world* property, and the bragging rights that come with it.

At one point, a major property developer in Dubai was building luxury condos that were marketing the promise of underwater views from every bedroom, living room, and kitchen. Yes! The condo was built into the ground, facing the Persian Gulf. Absolute decadence, right? But the kicker was this... as an extra incentive for each new home buyer, the property came with a bonus of a free, brand-spanking-new Ferrari—the only caveat was that it could only be in red.

If you've got the money, you can buy a luxury condo with the click of a finger, and move in the next week. But no matter how much money you have, you can't get your hands on a brand new Ferrari right away. You've got to be vetted, and there's at least a one-year waiting list before your baby gets delivered.

People were buying the condos...for the Ferrari!

Here's my point...Sometimes your client or customer will end up buying your product because of the amazing bonus they get with it. So keep that in mind. Don't just package junk bonuses together with your product...it has to have true utility value to the customer, and it is only then that you are truly giving your customer "the long end of the stick"...and you will be rewarded.

Now that you have a firm grip on finding your attractive character, and defining your brand and platform for your voice, you need to eventually develop a system and portfolio of products to make money. The way businesses get to market these days is just amazing, and you need to understand why, by taking a deep dive into what I call, *Middle-Man Money*.

See you on the next page...

# Chapter 5

# Middleman Money


*"The best investment you can make is an investment in yourself...
the more you learn, the more you'll earn."*
– Warren Buffet

## Supermarkets and the China Boom

I remember when I was a kid growing up in a middle class neighborhood in Hong Kong, during the 1970s and 1980s. I had an extended circle of acquaintances, which included several *businessmen*.  We all had one thing in common: tennis. I was a top junior player and competed internationally for the Hong Kong national team. Everyone in my circle wanted to beat me, including men 15 years older.

These businessmen wanted to play the game like I played it, and I got an early insight into the world of business back then, when China was just starting to open its borders to trading with the rest of the world.

A couple of guys, who I really got to know well, just wanted to talk about money, making deals, and girls. I didn't have a girlfriend back then, and I was already in my mid-teens (okay, so I was a late-bloomer). But they introduced me to the world of *middleman money.*

As China was opening up trade to the world, with cheap factory labour, North American companies were looking to expand, and to acquire low cost resources like garments, water pipes, steel, iron ore, electronic components, wiring, semiconductors...just about anything you named, the West wanted it at low cost. China was the answer.

The only problem was that Corporate America didn't have contacts in China. The likes of Motorola, JCPenney, The Gap, Neiman Marcus, Sears...were all gunning for a piece of the China boom in low-cost resources. This trade boom positioned Hong Kong uniquely as the gateway into China.

My friends became conduits and took commissions between the American buyers and suppliers in China. This was middleman money in its purest form.

All commission-based businesses play the middleman money game. Middleman companies merely connect, and don't have any products of their own. They offer a service. Middlemen rely on their expertise, network of contacts, and negotiation skills.

Middleman money is as old as commerce. Recruitment agencies are in the middleman money game. They connect companies, looking to hire, with people looking for a job.

If you look at its most basic form, middleman businesses are all around us: convenience stores, supermarkets, Walmart, 7-Eleven. The basic business model is: rent a huge warehouse, put in a whole bunch of shelves, and make money selling products from other companies. All these supermarkets have to do is to get customers into the store.

I had a client in Singapore, who invested a lot of money in creating their own dietary supplements but didn't know how to get them to market. Products were stocked in a warehouse, and it was costing them money. They decided to learn all about how to market their business online, by learning and starting an affiliate marketing business. This type of business model teaches you how to take an idea and attract leads, and how they convert into customers.

When I asked this mother-daughter partnership why they wanted to learn affiliate marketing (becoming a middleman with marketing other companies' products for a commission), they said why not start learning how to market other people's products in order to take this skill set back into their business.

Pretty smart.

## Leverage Other People's…Then Go Build Your Own

There are literally hundreds of different ways that you can start a business and generate cash flow. Rather than trying to list out everything, I thought it would be more valuable to teach you some fundamental lenses through which you need to assess some important strategic principles of how you approach your business.

My guess is that you're not looking to make hobby income, for which there are hundreds of different ways to do it online. But you have a big idea in mind, and I'll bet you're looking to build a significant size business to impact a large number of people in your marketplace.

So, here are the five entrepreneur lenses, and master skills sets on how to plan out your business, before we get into the technical side of lead generation and customer conversion systems:

**#1: Build a turn-key business operation**: Have systems in place for your business so that the business runs without it owning you. When you have people and systems selling for you in your business, you have bought yourself time and financial freedom.

**#2: Outsourcing**: This frees up your time. Delegate and outsource repetitive tasks to someone else, and get experts to save you time from figuring it out all by yourself. I used to love doing everything myself. Learn the "how," but then delegate someone else to do the job. You'll know enough not to be robbed by over-inflated fees and longer than necessary lead times.

When you combine a turn-key business operation and outsourcing that does the selling for you, you are well on the way to true wealth creation: cash flow while preserving your time.

**#3: Paid advertising**: This is the quickest and most effective way to grow your business. We'll get into this later in the chapter. If you're impatient, there are only 3 number metrics you need to know to start running and scaling your business. (Just flip through toward the end of the next chapter, and I'll show you what these 3 numbers are.)

**#4: Invest in a mentor or a coach, or ideally, both.** You need someone in your corner who has been through the typical traps and mistakes, so that you can save time and money by avoiding them. Mentors instilled in me the importance of writing good copy, and learning the speak-to-many skillset, which compressed my time and scaled my personal development and revenue growth. And that's how I became an international lead speaker and trainer, and how I have created marketing funnels that converted over 35% of every visitor that landed on my web page.

**#5: Attend masterminds and workshop events** so that you're learning while networking. Chances are that you'll meet a guru that will give you one insight that took them years to discover, which could launch or take your business to another level. I learned the power of joint venture partnerships, and met my first JV partner as a result of attending a mastermind.

Depending on how you learn, you might start with working with an already proven system of selling to the extent that you can design a system for your own business further down the road.

The best way to learn how a business runs itself through systems is by taking a look at the job you're currently in right now. Pay particular attention to:

1) how the company find leads and prospects
2) how the company converts them into customers
3) how the product is delivered and fulfilled
4) how the company sets up its customer service and support
5) how the company sells more to that same customer

This is the most critical system workflow that any business must have in place, because it deals with revenue and cash flow. Everything else you can outsource: legal, accounting, hiring, IT systems.

You can also learn and work on a business that already has a selling system setup, without much risk.

Take network marketing as an example. You may be the type, like me, who hates selling to friends and family, and losing them in the process. I got into network marketing for about 18 months, because I wanted to learn the system for selling an idea.

Affiliate marketing, internet marketing, direct response marketing...it's referred to as different names, but it all means the same thing. It's a middleman business model that essentially connects the buyer with a seller of a product, and you take a commission of the transaction. The majority of the most profitable internet marketing business models deals with information and training products in digital form. The margins are huge, which explains why the commission payouts are big too—because there's no reproduction cost, no delivery or distribution cost, and the fulfillment and customer support is done 100% by the company, not you. The beauty of affiliate marketing, within the longer-term view of building your own business idea, is that it will teach you how to market an idea online through funnels, social media, email marketing, search engine optimization (SEO), and everything else involved, to get somebody, halfway around the world, to buy a product that you don't even own, for which you make a commission.

The current big trending middleman business model is in e-commerce, specifically the *drop shipping model*. Step 1) You create and host an online store, using a lot of easy-to-use platforms out there that have a drag-and-drop method. Step 2) You find products made in China, and you get them to make, store, and fulfill the orders directly to your customers. Step 3) You mark up the cost of the product, and you sell at over 5 times. Step 4) Run advertising to your store for people to buy, and the order gets sent directly to the factory and delivered to the doorstep of your customer. Step 5) You keep the profit between the sales price minus the cost of the product and delivery expenses.

The best but most expensive business model to get into, to learn selling and marketing, is franchising—McDonald's being the most famous business franchising model ever created. Regardless of the size format of the restaurant, it is the operating manual that makes the McDonald's business model work so efficiently, all around the world. Franchises work off of turn-key operations that are independent of the business owner showing up to work.

These are just a few extremely powerful examples, where you can learn how to build systems around your business; but as you're learning through these business models, you can make money on the side, as you work on building out your own business idea.

Without beating a dead horse, I must reiterate that having a turn-key system in place for your business is the most critical way to generate revenue.

That's rooted in the power of having an effective marketing funnel.

## The Anatomy of a Marketing Funnel

In the previous chapter, I gave you a short, simple overview of why your business needs a funnel (or several funnels). Now let's take a deep dive into the anatomy of a funnel, in an easily digestible form.

Funnels have always existed. The original AIDA Model (Awareness-Interest-Decision-Action) was developed by the big advertising agencies on Madison Avenue, as a way to explain a system of how a company should advertise and sell its products and services.

Mass media, through TV, radio, print, and outdoor billboards, gets a lot of people into the stores to buy. While a lot of this has been replaced by more relevant advertising channels, the principles remain.

Today, we no longer search for stuff in the Yellow Pages but via Google; we watch less television but entertain ourselves on YouTube; and we find out about the world via Facebook.

Your business must encompass at least one, if not all, of three top social channels today: Google, YouTube, and Facebook (or Instagram, which is also owned by Facebook, in case you didn't know). If you're not in or considering using any of these channels in your future business, you are missing out on a whole lot customers, as well as system efficiency in finding them.

So, let's get into the anatomy of a funnel and how each step works.



Copyright© Ian Billingham, 2019.

Starting from the left side, which is the *entrance* to your marketing and selling funnel system:

You always want to show your ad, and target your spending to the right kind of people, who are most likely going to buy a product. That's called targeting. The purpose of an ad is to filter out likely buyers from those who will never buy, which is the next step in the funnel, called *qualifying*. Now you want to educate these leads on your offer and its benefits. This is the process of how your business engages with your lead or prospect to move them one step closer to a buying decision.

Once you've got their attention, now is the time to ask for the sale. This is when you convert that prospect into a paying customer, and money comes into your company's pockets.

That's a fundamental breakdown of how a funnel works. Unfortunately, your business can't depend on just one funnel. Your gut is probably telling you that you're going to need several different types of funnels. You're right. You'll want to cast the widest net out there to attract leads, and use different methods in the conversion cycle, as people need to be convinced by different means, and may need longer or shorter times before making a decision.

Now you need to determine how to get your advertising messages out there so that human beings will click on those messages and ads, and end up landing on the first page or first step of your funnel. This is called traffic. Traffic is people.

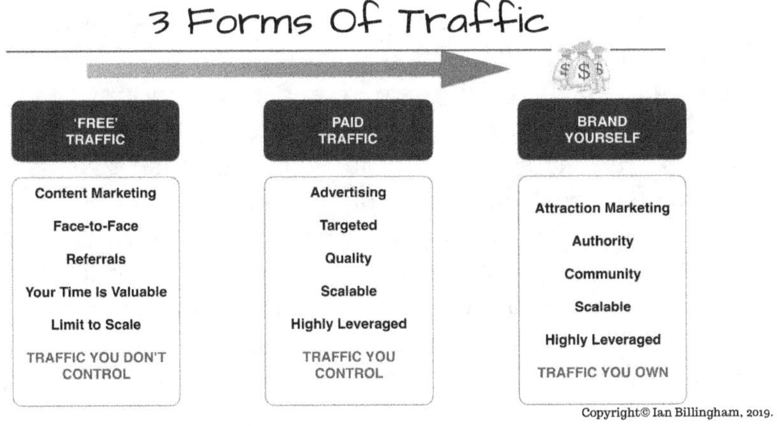


Copyright© Ian Billingham, 2019.

There are three forms of traffic, and if I can at least educate you at a minimum on what to watch out for, as internet gurus are likely going to confuse you with contradicting information, then I've done my job in helping you make a clear decision on the kind of traffic strategy that's right for your business.

Free traffic is essentially not paying money for advertising to get people to go to your site. This can be through writing a blog, creating a video on YouTube, meeting face to face with your prospects, or getting referrals from colleagues, family, and friends. This method doesn't cost money, but it costs you time, and time is money. Since you cannot scale time, this traffic is very difficult to get large numbers of leads continuously into your funnel. You also can't control this type of traffic, and you're basing your business on the hope and prayer that somebody you meet, or accidentally lands on your blog or video, ends up buying from you. There is no such thing as free traffic, because the time it takes to create the content, or meet a prospect, costs you money. Your time is money.

Paid traffic or paid advertising is scalable, and it's the type of traffic to your business that you can control. In many advertising platforms, on Google, Facebook, Instagram, Snapchat, Twitter, LinkedIn, or Pinterest, you can tell these platforms exactly what you want to show, where you want to show it, to whom you want to show it, when in the day, and what amount of spend you want to budget for. You get instant hourly feedback on how your ads are performing, so that you can make tweaks and adjustments in real-time. As soon as you know that your ad is working (meaning lots of people are seeing your ads, lots of people are clicking, lots of people are opting in, and some of them are starting to buy your product), that's when you can start to scale and grow your business by putting in more advertising, and boosting the reach and intensity of your campaigns.

I'll cover more on scaling and growing your business, in the next chapter.

But the ultimate traffic is the traffic you own. Over a period of time, you will have acquired a database of leads and prospects because of the ad campaigns that you've been running. Your database can be a list of names and email addresses from your opt-in pages, a Facebook Fan Page or Instagram following, a community of newsletter subscribers, etc... If there is a way you can reach out and contact these leads and prospects again, you now own and control your traffic. But since you've already paid for this traffic, you can now market to them over and over and over again, without paying any additional ad spend. This is when you can direct that database traffic anywhere you choose in your business.

Your most important equation to understand how you are marketing your business online is this:

## The Most Important Funnel Equation

## [Quality] Traffic + Conversions = Sales

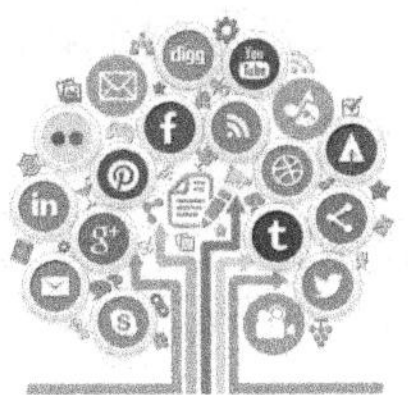 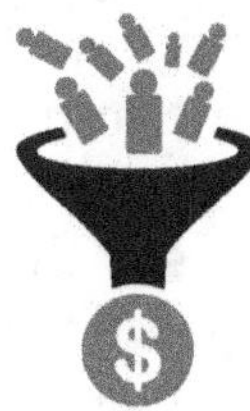 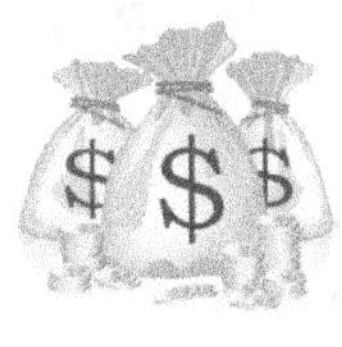

Your business makes money when you have the right people seeing your ads, becoming leads, and then converting into paying customers. It is a number's game. Focus on the conversion side; the traffic will come relatively easily.

At the end of this chapter, I'm going to reveal to you your single biggest asset that will make you money for life. Just hang in there, as there are some other fundamentals you need to grasp...

## You're Guaranteed to Lose Money on Your First Offer

Chances are that your first business idea isn't going to be selling massive heavy machinery that costs hundreds of thousands of dollars. More likely, your first business will include a product or service priced very affordably, like a smart device, a supplements jar, a nutritional product, a gym membership, a coaching program, an online training program, or even a book.

Business fact: You will lose money every time you sell this to your first-time customers, because of your customer acquisition cost.

Let me illustrate this by using the revenue model from the most famous Scottish restaurants of all time: McDonald's.

On the next page is a simplified diagram of McDonald's multi-billion dollar revenue generating marketing funnel.

From all their data analysis, they know that it takes $1.91 in advertising to get someone through the drive-thru or into the restaurant, who will spend, on average, $2.09—this is called the *front end* of the funnel. McDonald's stands to profit $0.18 by subtracting marketing and advertising costs from the average revenue per customer on their first purchase. Doesn't sound like a lot, does it? Well, it gets more interesting...

## McDonald's Funnel Model

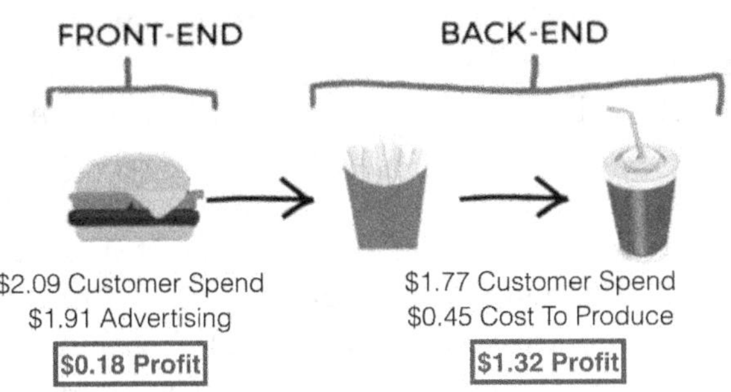




When was the last time you went to a McDonald's restaurant? And what's the typical question you get from the cashier when you put in your order? (Now, this is back in the old days, before self-service kiosk machines halved the required staff to run a McDonald's outlet.)

*"Would you like a drink with that? How about some fries?"* And if you really want to go further back in time (as it's banned in several countries now), *"Would you like to supersize that?"*

This is McDonald's upsell. They are getting you to buy more...and they know you will.

Since they've already profited from getting you through the drive-thru or into the restaurant, anything else you buy with the burger will be mostly profit. By *upselling* you the fries and coke, for which you'll pay an additional $1.77—and they know the cost of producing the fries and coke is roughly $0.45—they stand to profit an additional $1.32 just with the upsell, for a total profit per customer of $1.50 ($0.18 on the *front end,* plus $1.32 on the *back end,* or upsell).

Apple, given their company size, has a surprisingly small portfolio range, but add in the different variations and technical configurations, they can offer a wide range across a small portfolio line-up. Apple stores are a mecca for millions and millions of people around the world. But it wasn't always like that. Sure, Apple still spends a lot of money on advertising to lure new customers and to switch customers from other competitive brands. So they know the amount of advertising it takes to get someone into a physical or online store to buy their first Apple product. Business economics dictates that they are likely going to lose money or, at best, break even on the sale to a first-time customer. They also know that over the lifetime of that customer, they will earn many, many times more, because you're going to come back and buy more stuff from Apple.

As you develop your product offering, you need to price each of your products or services strategically, so that, 1) you offer a product your customer can experiment with; 2) you cross-sell or up-sell your customer to buy complementary products; 3) you gear your product offering so that your customers come back and buy again; and 4) you offer something for special customers, who are looking to buy something even more extraordinary, and are prepared to pay a very high price for it.

Because of the advertising dollars required to send traffic to your funnel, a small percentage of your leads will end up being your customers. Economics dictates that you will lose money on your first-time buyers.

Your profits, however, are made on the back end. It works when you can upsell them into a higher performing product or service, enroll them into a subscription, or get them to come back and buy again. That's when you start making profits off of that same customer, because you have already absorbed the advertising cost to acquire that customer in the first place.

This is called escalating your customer up your value ladder.

I take the clients that I teach, who have not mapped out their product ladder yet, or who have one but are not making any money from it yet, through my *BrandQ Value Ladder Blueprint*™.

And this is what it looks like.

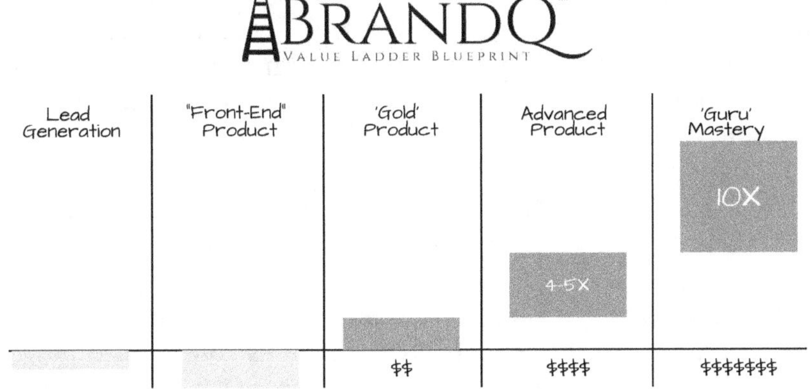


You spend time and advertising dollars to get people into your funnel. In exchange for their name and email address, you offer them something that is of value and is free: a lead magnet. You haven't made any money yet, because people haven't bought anything. This is your lead generation phase.

As you spend money to nurture these leads, and more advertising dollars to widen your net, some will end up buying your *front end* product. The revenue you get from the sale of your front end product will unlikely be enough to recoup your marketing expense, so you actually end up losing money on the front end.

A good proportion of these first-time customers are likely going to be funneled into buying your *Gold Product,* typically priced at a few hundred dollars. This could also be in the form of a subscription service model, with recurring monthly payments. You'll start to recoup more of your marketing expense, and may even start turning a small profit.

A small proportion of these customers will want more from you as they are beginning to trust you and would consider something more advanced that you could offer them. Your next level product is typically priced 4 to 5 times more than your Gold Product. This is the stage where you are starting to generate profits, especially if you have very low product and fulfillment costs. Typically, digital training products are the best, as the margins are huge, without the associated costs of fulfillment.

The ultimate product is to upsell and offer an exclusive *guru-*master type of product, priced 10 times more, with much more profit. This would depend on your product niche. In the business coaching and consulting niche, this could be private mentoring and a form of one-to-one access to you, the expert.

Remember, marketing is a numbers game: You will have tens of thousands of people coming into the first step of your funnel, starting from the left side of the graph, and less than 5% will be a top-paying client.

Hopefully, by now, you understand that you're not going to make any money with just offering front end products, because of the cost of your marketing. The real money is made on your upsell, or what you can additionally offer to your customers who will gladly pay you a lot more money for your best high performance product or service.

This value ladder is the basis for any product portfolio, regardless of whether it is a physical product, consumer or industrial goods product, subscription software, or a professional coaching or consulting service.

If you're looking to build a business based on your expertise, your intellectual property, your experience, and your skillset, then the *BrandQ Value Ladder Blueprint* is what you'll need to create and roll out into the marketplace.

## Your Single Biggest Asset That Will Pay You for Life

Your fortune is in your list.

In a report by MailMunch, 2016, they reported that "...email marketing drives more conversions than any other marketing channel, including social and search" (source: Monetate).

This is because, with the help of many software platforms and email service providers now, you can deliver highly targeted messages based on the behavior of your subscribers.

I know what you might be thinking: "Email ...what? ...didn't that go away with dial-up internet connection?"

Well, here's the reality that might surprise you. Maybe not everyone is still on email; but the majority of your potential customers are.

Then, why?

When somebody gives you their best email—and there are techniques to extract someone's preferred email address— they're giving you access to their private world. It's like opening the front door to their home.

Email is the best source of new and repeat traffic, where you can direct your subscribers to your blog, your video, other sections of your website, products, new launches, your training programs, or your upsells. You've already paid for the traffic to acquire the lead, so anything that you direct that subscriber to do, doesn't cost you anything additional.

Your subscriber list is like owning your very own piece of real estate in the cloud, which will make you money for life.

When somebody opens their email on desktop, or reads it on their phone, there's nothing else to distract them. Your email literally occupies their entire screen!

It takes less than 30 minutes to write an email, but you never have to spend the time to write that same email again. So, you can leverage that one time effort to make you money, over and over again. The best email marketers will reveal that you can expect to earn roughly $1 per subscriber per month, in your business. At one stage, I came close to $0.72 per subscriber per month.

An email message has the longest lifespan out of any other medium. That's because that email, read or unread, sits in your subscribers inbox until they open it. I've seen many participants, in a room full of entrepreneurs, who invested in a $30,000 program, confess that they had been receiving consistent email messages from the guru on stage, for the past 3 years, before they eventually bought. Three years as a lead before becoming a customer...because of email!!

Be patient.

And the best thing about a subscriber list is that it's a transferable asset for your other businesses. You could be marketing and selling one product or service today, but because you've built up a reputation, and trust and connection with your community or list (just refer back to the chapter on You Inc.), they will follow you into your new business, which could be completely unrelated to the reason why they subscribed to you in the first place.

Your email list is therefore your biggest money-making asset, for you and for your business, because building an email list is like building a human relationship with your community.

A subscriber database can be your email list; it can be thousands of your Instagram followers, followers of your Facebook Fan Page, people in your Facebook group, or on your newsletter...all your list needs to have to enable you to reach out to them is some form of communication channel for you to engage with them, and in turn, be influenced by you to take them somewhere in your funnel that will deliver them value.

The next chapter is on a topic that you've probably been waiting for. How do you market online with social media? How does it work? Should I use Facebook or Twitter? What's the best social media platform to use? How should I use social media in my business?

I'm going to break this down, so turn the page, and let's get started.

# Chapter 6

# Social Media: That's All Greek to Me

*"What we've got here is a failure to communicate."*
– The captain's speech (*Cool Hand Luke*, 1967)

## It's All One Big Giant Party!

I've got good news and bad news. Which would you like first?

The good news?

The good news is that all social media works. The bad news is that all social media works.

You need to figure out what works for you.

I'm an introverted guy. I like my alone time. I'm actually quite shy, and I freeze up when I enter a room full of people. When I started my new career, after I left the corporate business world, networking was an essential part of the game plan. If you're like me, you're probably going to appreciate some battle proven insights and advice I'm going to share with you on how to survive and thrive in the business networking world, and walk away with a stack of business cards and contacts.

Arrive early, and head for the bar. Nobody likes to walk into a room full of people who are already deep into the second or third round of conversation. It's awkward introducing yourself to a group that's already engrossed in discussing the latest fake news, last night's fight, and cat videos. Everyone heads to the bar to get their first drink, so if you're already there, you're in line of sight for somebody else to introduce themselves to you...first. You also get the best vantage point, from the bar, to strategically scan the floor.

Establish your small group early. Everybody likes to join a conversation with a small group. Large groups are too intimidating. The trick is to attract people to you; if the other person is entering your group, social etiquette dictates that they have to make the first introduction. Now, doesn't that take the stress off your shoulders?

Once you've got your own group started, you can begin to navigate the room and meet other people. It's so much easier. If there's a group that you've spotted from your eagle-eye vantage point at the bar, or you've spotted someone you'd like to meet, who is looking a little awkward (because they didn't buy *The Big Shift* and take my advice on networking), grab a couple people from your group and begin the approach. Security and power comes in numbers; make sure it's working for you and not against you.

Bring name cards, but also be prepared to exchange your social media contacts. This gives you the option of handing over a business card at the end of a more formal introduction to somebody that you want to keep in touch with, or use your phone to share your contact details with somebody with whom you socially connected with. It's all about having options and ammunition in social networking warfare.

Social media is exactly like real life social networking...on steroids.

What Facebook, Pinterest, Instagram, Snapchat, WeChat, and Tumblr all have in common is what I'm about to tell you. It's going to help demystify all the technological *mumbo jumbo* with what it's going to take to get leads, prospects, and customers online.

It's all a party.

Social media is just one...giant...global...PARTY!!

It's a house full of different groups of like-minded individuals, talking about common things and interests: the *in* crowd, the *out* crowd, the geeks, the nerds, the jokers, and groups of people that create their own group because they don't want to belong to any group—huh??

As a newcomer to the party, you've got to figure out where and how to introduce yourself.

The best way to find out is to figure out what shared interests you have with them. It's connecting what you have to offer, in line with the values of the audience group.

But be warned:  The first thing that comes out of your mouth, or post, could either get you immediately accepted into their inner circle, get you kicked off, or have you cast out to the fringes, where you have to work your way back in, slowly and carefully.

Once you understand the basic psychology—that social media is like one giant party—you can start making inroads like you would do in real life.

My golden rule: If you wouldn't do it in real life, don't do it online.

## Breaking Down Basics

The over-eagerness of any new business owner, who's just starting out marketing their product on social media, is to start pitching right at the get go.

Let's use the analogy of the real life party again.

Would you ever start passing out name cards and pitching your business right at the moment you walk into a social gathering? When you're invited for the first time to somebody's house, do you automatically go straight to the sofa, put your feet on the coffee table, and start criticising the host's bad taste in curtains? No, of course not.

So, why would you start pitching your business as soon as you get on social media?

Social media changes all the time, and they have built and continue to augment their data algorithms and artificial intelligence and robots to understand how people react and behave online. Whatever social media platform that's the *in thing* these days, there are three basic fundamentals that don't change much when marketing online, and I learnt this from one of my business partners, who's an ex-Facebook employee and has worked in the global marketing department.

Engage; consider; convert—and it has to be in that order.

The old AIDA advertising model hasn't fundamentally changed much: Get people AWARE of your idea; then INFORM them of the features and benefits of your product; lead your prospects to a DECISION; and then get them to take ACTION to go to their local store and buy.

Engaging your audience on social media is like dating. It's about joining a conversation, making some smart comments, and finding the opportune time to introduce yourself. If you're interesting enough, you'll get questions, and that's when it'll slowly pave the way to share more of your back story. Early dates are like feeling each other out, and figuring out if there's going to be a second date. What this looks like is when they are starting to like, comment, and share your posts.

The phase when your social community is starting to consider you is when you begin the education part of your story or business. They're saying, "Hey Ian, I like what you said. Can you tell me more about this?" It's when you're adding variety to your relationship, buying chocolates, and making sweet promises you don't intend to keep (now which movie is that line from??). They're clicking on your post, sharing, making comments, and checking out your website.

The final stage is the conversion phase.

Now, this could be any number of things, depending on what you want your community to be doing next. This is called the action: clicking on a link to find out more about a new website; subscribing to newsletters; opting in to attend a webinar training; watching a video; adding something to cart; downloading an app; or even buying your product because of a special time-sensitive discount offer. Whatever that *conversion* is, it can only be established once you've engaged your audience, and after they've gone through a process of considering what you have to say.

You'd never pop *the question* on the first or second date, would you?

Conversion can take weeks, or it can take months. It all depends on what you want to achieve, and how well you have done on the previous *engaging* and *considering* stages.

It also varies by industry niche.

For example, the process of buying a new property from a real estate agent that you don't even know, could take some time. Buying a new software that does things a lot better than an older version, takes arguably a little bit less time. Buying a candle with an amazing new fragrance, at a 50% discount, wouldn't take much time at all.

If you don't get these basics right, and have the patience to go through these necessary steps, you'll end up being frustrated and ready to give up. You might end up creating ads that constantly pitch and annoy the social media community, because you want people to buy now.

If you're on Facebook, you're likely going to have your Facebook ad account shut down, which means you can no longer advertise campaigns; or your ads will not get approved immediately; or your ads are not being delivered by Facebook well, and you end up wasting a lot of money.

To use the house party analogy again, it's like getting to the party, having a few too many drinks, and you still haven't found a girlfriend or boyfriend, and you get desperate and start acting obnoxiously. The party host gets informed, and the entire house goes into emergency shut down mode on you. House security races in with pepper spray, and throws you out the door.

You either shape up or ship out.

So, respect the social media platform, and follow Engage, Consider, and Convert...in that order.

## Fundamentals and Secret Cheats

Because social media platforms change their algorithms all the time, and data processing and data-mining activities are geared to improving the overall user experience (which is their multi-billion dollar *Holy Grail*), I'm not about to teach you the step-by-step manual on how to do this and how to do that, because chances are, by the time this book gets out, everything will have changed.

Instead, I'm going to teach you the key principles.

Tactics always change; principles stick.

I'm going to give you one starting fundamental principle before you start any social media marketing...

Trust.

Every post you send out into the world, whether it be a message, a photo, a blog or a story, you are opening yourself up to the world of criticism and cynicism. Let's assume for just a moment that your post passes the thumb swipe test (that's when people are *thumbing* through their news feed, and stop to check out a post), and suddenly, your post is the only thing the reader sees on their phone. That's already a big milestone achieved.

Once a viewer pauses on your post, chances are they're going to check out your profile, or if you post it through a Facebook fan page, they're going to want to check out how many followers and likes you have. It's the trust factor test.

They're checking to see if you're legit, and who you are.

And that, unfortunately and superficially, is about how many followers you have, in the case of Instagram, and how many likes you have on your Facebook fan page. (I'm using examples on these platforms as they are the biggest...and both are owned by Facebook.)

Starting a new business will require getting instant credibility and trust (at a basic level). I'm going to reveal a secret cheat to get you thousands of likes on your Facebook Fan Page in a week...with just a few bucks.

Create a fan page, and then create your first post—ideally, a post of a picture with some catch phrase. Then create a *Likes* campaign behind it, and target that post to be shown to people in the following countries, selecting English as a language preference: India, Philippines, and Indonesia (there are a few more countries, but try these to start). Set aside a campaign budget for 7 days, for about $40, and then, within a week, you'll have several thousand likes on your Fan Page. Facebook users in these countries just love pressing the *Like* button on just about anything—it's a cultural social thing. And it only costs you less than a penny per *Like*.

Boom—instant credibility!

But don't overdo it. Just give it a small burst. If you do it too often, you'll likely have problems with placing ads, and it will take longer to get your ads approved, or your ads won't deliver well. Facebook police might think there's something fishy with your fan page.

My buddy, Dr. Roger (and he is a real doctor, and that's his real name), built his Instagram following to over 50,000 followers, in under 8 months. I dragged him on stage once to teach a class of business owners how he did it. He gave the performance of a lifetime; the audience was hanging on every word he was saying, and he was absolutely in his element.

I want to share these 9 secrets from the notes I took while sitting at the back of the room:

#Secret1: Don't switch between personal/business accounts (because you have both in Instagram); stick with one for good engagement.

#Secret2: Use business accounts to *boost*, via paid ads, and get post analytics.

#Secret3: Use multiple accounts for multiple brands, if you have multiple businesses.

#Secret4: Always use quality hashtags that are congruent with your post; select hashtags with 10,000 to 1 million posts, as those conversations are indicative of starting or trending.

#Secret5: Put hashtags in comments immediately AFTER the post, not within the post's text. This was an algorithm change in Instagram, back in 2016.

#Secret6: Add new people just starting out: They will stick with you, as they also want to build their own following.

#Secret7: DM (direct message) to big influencers in your niche: pay to get *shout out/featured*.

#Secret8: Four posts per day: morning wake-up, lunch, after work, before bed.

#Secret9: Hashtags and location where you're posting from gets more views/engagement.

Got an Instagram account?  Start trying these out, and let me know how you're getting on.

## Your Business Flourishes on Just These 3 Numbers

Numbers and key performance indicators (KPI) are the eyes and ears of your business. They are the GPS compass that tells you the velocity and direction you're heading in with your business, so that you can make some very important investment decisions and know where to focus, fix, and scale.

I've worked in enough companies to know the obsession with numbers. Three or four times a year, we would have massive corporate presentations on the business, and would spend weeks creating hundreds of PowerPoint slides, including backups of backups, and reams and reams of data, just on the off chance that the *big dogs* asked a question about a data point, and we would be ready to answer it.

In the real world of entrepreneurship, especially in the early stages, there's really only a few numbers that actually matter, outside of cash flow.

We've already covered the anatomy of a funnel and how it works, so these three key metrics are essentially the most critical funnel stages that tell you how efficient you are with your marketing investments and cash-flow:

**Lead Conversion Rate (LCR):** This is a measure of how many people out of 1000, who clicked on your ad and landed on the first page at the start of your funnel, submitted their name and email address details, and became a lead in your database. Leads are an important flow into your business as over time they become paying customers. Your opt-in page or lead-generation page must convert at no less than 30%; meaning, out of 1000 people, 300 of them enter their name and email addresses. I've built lead conversion funnels that convert close to 40%, and I use this as the basis to build my client's lead generation funnels.

**Customer Acquisition Cost (CAC):** This is the total advertising and marketing spend for a given period of time, divided by the number of paying customers of your front end product.

Let's say your front end product retails for $100; you spend $1,500 in advertising, and you acquire 5 customers of your product. Your cost to acquire each customer is $300 — you spent $1,500 in advertising and only got $500 in revenue, so you're in the hole for $1,000. But if you know that 20% of your customers will go on to buy a $2,500 product (that's 1 customer out of the 5 you just got from this example), you've now made $1,500 net profit ($500 + $2,500, minus advertising of $1,500). So, in this case, your cost to acquire a customer can actually be much higher than the price of your front end product — and that's ok — so long as you know that you've got a much higher priced product that you can upsell your customer, and you know how your funnel converts.

This is where you make money. So long as you know your customer acquisition cost, and you set that as a threshold, you now have a lot more confidence in the way you spend your advertising, because your advertising and funnel is making you money, and you can now look for other ways to further improve.

**Average Customer Lifetime Value (ACLV):** This is calculated by taking a period of time, usually anywhere from six months to a year, and dividing your total revenue by the number of paying customers you have in that period. The significance of the ACLV measure is that it tells you the maximum amount of advertising that you can spend to acquire a customer. You will know that within six months to a year, you will generate this amount back on a per customer level...your average break-even point.

This is what the big consumer household brands, like Apple, Samsung, and Kellogg's, will do to dominate the marketplace. The company that dominates the marketplace is the one who is prepared to spend the most to acquire a customer—more than any of their competitors.

## One Dollar In; Two Dollars Out

The previous three metrics essentially tell you the life blood and cash flow of your business.

There is actually a 4th metric. It's the measure that determines when, and how quickly, you can start to scale your business.

**Advertising Return on Investment (AROI):** This is the return on investment (ROI) measure of how much advertising you put in, versus how much revenue comes out the other end. Using the previous example, you generated $3,000 in gross revenue on $1,500 ad spend. Your return on investment is 200%. Tell me an investment out there that can generate this level of return. Your business will get you to a level where you're likely spending thousands, if not tens of thousands, of dollars per day, because you know your ROI numbers. If your product sells on Amazon, then there's a slightly different measure on your ROI. Amazon uses *Advertising Cost of Sales* (ACOS): how much advertising was spent as a percentage of total gross sales revenue. This gives you a slightly different view of your ROI. If your ACOS is around 20%, then your ROI on sales is roughly 5 to 1: you spent $1 in advertising to get $5 in sales revenue. An ACOS target number will depend on your sales margin for the product you are selling on Amazon, usually at 15–17% of gross sales revenue. Whatever the number is, once you hit that target number, you have the first indications that your business has finally got some traction and is poised for growth.

So, how do you increase your revenue and business growth? Just spend more...once you know you're converting customers profitably.

Show your ad campaigns to more people. When you have a positive return on your ad spend, you can confidently spend more because you'll have enough revenue coming out the other end to at least cover your marketing cost.

One of the very first questions I was asked by my mentor was, "What's your ad budget?"

The general rule of thumb in the corporate world was roughly 2% of projected revenues. During the course of the year, your marketing budget would either go up or down, depending on whether the company was ahead or behind sales targets. Companies actually will limit or even cut the marketing spend if targets are not being met; while the flip side can sometimes happen when a company decides to invest more in marketing when performance is ahead of forecasts.

This is another mind shift you need to make as an entrepreneur. You can literally spend profitably with marketing your business online, using real-time analytics from all these social media marketing platforms.

If your campaigns are converting profitably for you, you should be spending as much as you can.

## Scaling

As soon as you know that more money is coming out the other end of your funnel than the ad spend you're investing in, you can begin to scale your revenues.

Unlike the old way of growing a business, the modern business doesn't need more stores, inventory, trucks, or employees. A predominantly internet-based way of marketing your business can have the potential to grow exponentially in a very short space of time.

Scaling a business online is purely about injecting more advertising dollars once you have profitable campaigns.

Here's a few quick ways to scale...

Enlarge your geographic reach. Advertising on social media platforms enables you to dictate exactly how wide, geographically, you want to show your ads. If these campaigns are converting profitably for you, and you're advertising only in, say, London, just by increasing your area by within a 50-mile radius around London could instantly get you more reach, leads, customers, and revenue. Then expand nationally to all of United Kingdom. Chances are that your demographics are pretty homogeneous within a given country, and it is highly likely that your funnels will continue to convert leads into customers profitably. More customers means more revenue.

The next level of geographic reach of your campaigns could be if you're advertising in the US, expand to another state or region, or go nationally; because the fundamental drive as to why people are reacting and converting in your campaigns is likely going to remain as you expand your campaigns across a broader geographical area. With some minor adjustments in copy tonality, headline, and image, you could quite quickly expand the reach of your campaigns, and scale your revenue quickly.

Expanding into new countries is another very quick way of scaling your business. If your product idea or service is principally English language based, then you have a number of choices of countries to expand the campaigns into: United States, Canada, United Kingdom, South Africa, India, Singapore, Hong Kong, Malaysia, Australia, and New Zealand.

Extending your campaigns into these markets may require some language modifications, as there could be slight language nuances and styles of speaking, which may have to be reflected in your campaign message.

If you are entering a new market, where English is not widely spoken, then you'll need to look into translation services. Amazon does this pretty well, and offers translation services for your product catalog and listings so that they appear in the local language in other Amazon marketplaces in Europe, like the United Kingdom, Germany, France, Italy, and Spain. Sometimes you may need to start new campaigns from scratch. But since you already have the experience of tweaking and testing campaigns to convert profitably, this should be a relatively smooth process.

By this stage, you should have already hired a digital marketing agency to run and manage all your social media campaigns.

Other ways to scale revenue is through pricing and product innovation or expansion.

If you can afford to make small increases in your product's pricing, then go for it.

Expanding your product portfolio ensures that you give your customers new reasons to come back and buy from you again.

But I'll save this for my next book.

So, now that you've got the basic mechanics of systems, funnels, marketing online with social media, and the numbers to focus on, I'm going to do a slight shift in the following chapters, and take you through the highest leveraged skill set, which you can learn simply by using an amazing tool that you were born with.

It's pretty advanced and will scare a lot of readers.

I'll see you in the next chapter.

# Chapter 7

# Million-Dollar Checkbook

*"The higher your energy level, the more efficient your body. The more efficient your body, the better you feel and the more you will use your talent to produce outstanding results."*
– Annie Lennox

## The Highest Leveraged Skill Set

People would rather die from drowning than speak in front of a crowd.

According to the 1977 edition of *The Book of Lists*, by David Wallechinsky, Irving Wallace, and Amy Wallace, "The 14 Worst Human Fears" put public speaking at the top of the list by a long shot. Here are the top 8 fears from the list:

- Public speaking
- Heights
- Insects and bugs
- Financial problems
- Deep water
- Sickness
- Death
- Flying

If you've been in the corporate world long enough, or the nature of your job requires you to attend a whole bunch of useless meetings or to lead a project team, then you will have had a chance to speak in front of an audience, however small. Congratulations, you've made the first cut!

Speaking is the most highly paid skill set there is, and as you will discover in this chapter, it's not a talent you're born with, but one that is perfected through training and experience. It is as much an art form as it is a science, as you'll find out.

Now, just so we're all on the same page, I'm not here talking about speaking in terms of lecturing, teaching, entertaining, or motivating for standing ovations or applauses, as these are disguised objectives of wanting to be popular or beloved.

I'm talking about speaking, where at the end of your speech, tens, hundreds, or thousands of people are rushing to the back of the room, credit card in hand, because they want to buy what you're selling.

I'm talking about speaking to sell—sometimes referred to as *platform selling*, or *selling from the stage*. So, to ease my poor fingers from typing out these labels every time, I'll just refer to this particular form, from now on, as *speaking*.

I got into speaking, purely by association with the right people. I had invested in some coaching and had 2 mentors at the time, who got me connected to companies looking to hire speakers to sell their products from the stage to large audiences. One of the company owners, who I had become close with, pulled me aside at a large conference in London, and asked me to walk with him to his car. He was on his way to the airport.

He knew I came from corporate, from a high level executive position, and had seen me on many occasions doing training from the stage. He explained where his company was heading, and by the time we reached his car, he already had his assistant book me on a flight the next day to head to Hong Kong. I was going on a reconnaissance, to observe what he was doing with events, and soon after, I became his lead speaker and trainer.

My first few events were a disaster. I knew how to speak, but my closing rate wasn't that good. I couldn't send people to the back of the room to buy the training I was selling. I couldn't close a door to save my life. But after a lot of careful feedback and analysis, I was soon touring with my own crew, speaking at free and paid events, and making a lot of money doing it.

I'll get to the structure of the kind of money you can expect to earn as a speaker, a little bit later in this chapter, but what it amounts to is this: You get a percentage of the total gross sales sold.

## Do This Each Day for 30 Days, and You're on Your Way to Speaker Hall of Fame

It's kind of ironic how I ended up speaking for a living, for multiple companies across four continents. The person who landed me my first speaking gig was the same person who got me to do this one trick a year earlier.

I believe now, in hindsight, he was grooming me to become his trainer and speaker.

A year earlier, I was given the challenge to do a video a day for 30 days straight, and I had to prove this by uploading them into my YouTube channel. My mentor, at the time, told me that only one of his clients had ever completed this challenge. So, being competitive by nature, I wanted to be next.

My first videos were an absolute joke. I averaged 23 takes to film a 4-minute piece on camera. Like anything in life, repetition produces progress, and progress produces results, and consistent results yields success.

I produced 30 videos in 30 days, and passed the challenge. But I wanted to keep going for another 30 days, and then another 60 days. I kept this up for 6 months, without interruption, and created a library of 170 videos on my YouTube channel, covering business, marketing, self-development, and entrepreneurship.

Filming in front of a camera, and just *yakking* away, comes quite naturally to me now. I only need one take to get it done; it doesn't have to be perfect, and whatever needs fixing can be done in post-editing. You know you've got it when you can pull out a magazine or newspaper article, or blog post, and ad-lib a 4-minute speech around that topic.

That was the activity and foundation that trained me how to verbalise, explain, and teach—but I wasn't a speaker just yet, as that was only a small part of the whole speaking science and art form.

## 4-Steps to 4-Minute Videos Formula

I just about perfected my process of video creation, and developed a simple system for you to start learning a structured way of organising your thoughts and delivering something in front of a camera.

I call it my *4-Steps to 4-Minute Videos Formula*, and here it is:

*The Intro*: Introduce yourself, and explain why the viewer should care. (This covers your brand and character from an earlier chapter.)

*The Pain Question*: Pose a question that's on the minds of your target audience.

*The Education*: Talk about your insight on the topic you're addressing.

*The Call-To-Action*: Tell the viewer what to do next.

So, to give an example of how it works, here's a typical video sequence that I use all the time to create my videos on my YouTube channel, with my brand, New Economy Wealth Secrets.

Here's my character and brand opening introduction:

> *Hey there, it's Ian Billingham, and welcome to another episode of New Economy Wealth Secrets, where I teach start-up business owners how to create, market, and monetize their business idea online.*

...here's the pain question:

> *Do you have a funnel for your business? Know what it is? Or are you super-confused with all the jargon the so-called gurus are teaching you?*

...here's Step-3, teaching the solution:

> *I get that question a lot from teaching start-up business owners...simply put, a funnel is a step-by-step process..... [and then, for 2–3 minutes,  I go on and explain*

*what a funnel is all about in simple terms,*
*and I may tell a story to make their learning more interesting]*

And now Step 4, the Call-To-Action:

*If you enjoyed that marketing tip for the day, and you're looking to*
*learn more, just click on the blue google link below this video,*
*and it'll take you to a page that will explain how you can get*
*my funnel training in 4 easy steps.*

*Subscribe to my channel if you liked it, and see you on the*
*next video for more insightful business and marketing tips from*
*New Economy Wealth Secrets. I'm Ian, signing off for now*
*...continued success to you!!*

That was simple, wasn't it?

Going from YouTube sensation to speaking on the stage is a long process, because there's an art and a science behind it. In a way, it is a performance, but not to be confused with an act.

Speaking is about influencing your audience to move one step closer to pulling out their credit card and buying what you're selling. Speaking has nothing to do with your ability to talk, and it's a skill that is learned. You must delicately navigate them through a journey of pain, emotion, hope, logic, and learning.

## Nine Secrets from the Stage

There are some fundamental structures and principles you need to have in place to be an effective speaker, and to get paid lots for doing what you love. Here are my top-9 secrets from the stage.

For all intents and purposes, these secrets relate to you being the only lead speaker/trainer, for an event seminar format with 50 to 150 people in the room, which is different from a *pitch-fest*, where you are just one of many speakers on the stage, pitching one product after another, in your 90-minute slot.

These are the types of events that I particularly enjoy, because of the intimacy and rapport you can build with your audience in selling programs priced in the multiple five-figure price levels. Seminar events also bring in the highest per-head revenue; and hence, requires a vastly different skill set to influence a room over multiple days.

Secret#1: *The Stage Is Your Performance Zone.* Split the stage up into 4 parts: left, right, front, back. Use the back or rear of the stage to tell your stories, and the front to deliver content so that you are closer to the audience, even lowering yourself when you want to connect with them on a more personal level while emphasizing how your content relates to them. Anchor the audience to stage left (your left; audience's right) when you talk about negative things. It's a visual reminder of the pain area. Use stage right (audience's left) to anchor the participant's mind for positive elements like hope, success, results, and a picture of a better future. You also use the audience's left on anything where you educate content using logic. Never mix and match using either of stages left and stage right, as it will confuse the audience. Anchor your markers in the beginning, with right or left, and stick to them.

Secret#2: *The Speaker Is CEO of the Room.* The speaker decides the flow of content and the journey he wants to effectively take the audience on, over the duration of the event, ending with the close. He controls everything that happens in the room, including the temperature, which needs to be cool enough to get the audience to wear a sweater and stay awake. The CEO defines the objectives of each section in the schedule of the event, and designs the content accordingly. In all of my 3-day workshops, I made sure that my team were aligned to my objectives in setting out the content: Day 1 was identifying the room (who's in the room); Day 2's goal was selling; and Day 3's objective was to collect the money. Notice that the event objectives are like running a business...because it is. Then align all your content and your strategy, with achieving these objectives.

Secret#3: *Your Team Is Your Biggest Feedback Mechanism.* As a main event speaker, you will normally work with a team of people supervised by a manager. Your sales team handles the event logistics, meets and greets the guests, gives you an overall feeling and profile of the room, and closes sales for you. You must establish a single point of contact with the team manager, who's going to give you live feedback as to how the room is reacting, the vibe, certain things that you need to stress, and keeps you on time. Your manager is going to be your biggest ally in the room.

Secret#4: *Navigating the Room Builds Rapport.* It is so important to win trust, and that's everything that builds a successful event or not. Get down to the audience's level by walking around the room as you're delivering content. I think speakers who only remain on the stage, like a lecturer, are missing a huge important facet behind influencing the room psychology. The audience will buy when you have the right combination of connecting rapport on the ground, with authority coming from the stage.

Secret#5: *Use the Audience to Magnify Your Credibility.* I do a lot of this on day one when I'm getting to know the audience, and the audience is getting to know me, their trainer, for the next few days. The team during the meet and greet will have prompted you on a few individuals in the audience that you could identify in making a point during your training. As you navigate the floor, ask them the question where you're guaranteed the response you want. And always solicit positive and "yes" responses—it builds up positive energy in the room. Besides, the individual is going to feel privileged to be picked out by the guru, having their 2 seconds of fame. Your audience will back you up and edify your credibility with the audience.

Secret#6: *Learn to Tell Winning Stories*. Storytelling is a great way to get your point across, because teaching through stories is engaging and memorable, and it makes you human and gives you variety in your performance. Winning stories can even be jokes. As soon as you get the audience to laugh or give you a positive reaction to something you say, mark that joke or story repertoire, and keep using it over and over again. If it works, keep it. If it doesn't, trash it. One of my winning stories is my YouTube encounter with a fitness guru named Mike Chang, which you read about in an earlier chapter. But you have to see me live perform this story with all the voice effects and gestures—it always gets the audience in stitches. Yes, I'm definitely a goofball at heart.

Secret#7: *Duplication Is the Secret to Big Pay Days*. You need to be able to replicate your delivery, word for word—every nuance, every story, every joke, every physical action, the way you speak, every close— for every single event. If you always change the way you deliver, you can't improve, because you've changed so many things that you don't know what worked and didn't work. Video record your events, and analyse the process. You're only as good as your last event, and it's always about perfecting it. If you're closing the room with 15% of the people in the audience who end up buying, then ask yourself what went wrong. Identify the mistakes, get feedback from the team, and at the next event, implement those changes. When you start converting consistently at 20 to 25%, you're rock solid and reliable, and it only takes a few tweaks here and there to get your numbers up. My highest room conversion rate has been 67%, which matched the company's all-time record, and I've been pretty consistent, between 23 and 27%, on a free event format. But I've also had bomb days, where I converted a 200-person room at only 12%. I could have been slightly off my game, or the jokes weren't punchy enough, or the close wasn't strong enough...or it could have been purely because the audience was irritated because we started late. We had one over-subscribed event in Hong Kong, and had over 100 people who couldn't get in. We ran out of chairs, and a third of the room was standing in what little space was left in the back. Things happen. You shrug it off and move onto the next.

Secret#8: *Win the Permission to Sell*. An event series that I've been most experienced in is a free event to back-end workshop. People attend a free, 90-minute preview session, during which I pitch a $500 offer to attend a 3-day workshop that returns to the same city 2 to 3 weeks later. Full on training happens at the 3-day workshop, plus I offer the opportunity for the participants to invest in further programs. While a lot of people, who do end up buying, are a little over sensitive to the whole selling thing, they will forgive you if done right. I would consistently end my 3-day events with my students coming up to me to thank me for the amazing training and learnings they received. There would often be some remarks about the hard selling, but they said that was okay, as they still enjoyed the event. As long as you're selling with integrity, you can win the audience's permission to sell to them. If the audience is not complaining that you're over selling, you haven't done your job. It's all about the duality of dancing on the edge: an invisible line that divides over-selling and not doing enough. This is the difference between a successful event, or heading home to your family with nothing and not making rent.

It can back-fire, however…

I was attending a workshop, as a student, some time back (I'm always learning), when the *guru lost the room* on the final day of an event, which is *speaker talk* for saying that the room was turned off by the speaker, and refused to buy anything. The training product was terrific, but their teaching style was intimidating and arrogant, and as one audience member put it, "...it was like walking on eggshells the whole weekend." After several altercations with a few participants, the room turned. It was an expensive learning for the organisers, and hopefully a valuable one for the *guru*.

Secret#9: *Train Your Audience to Your Commands*. Train your audience to obey your commands, and they'll rush to the back of the room to buy from you. When you're speaking to sell, you want the audience to be on your side. Ask questions to the audience frequently, and get them to raise their hand in agreement with you. What you're actually getting them to do is not just agree with you, but you're training them to follow your commands. When the time comes, and you tell them to enroll in your programs by going to the back of the room to buy, they will. And this is a very skillful art that every speaker needs to master: Influence the audience to do what you want them to do.

So, how much money can you really make as a speaker? What's life like on the road? One of your nightmares is to be confronted by a troublemaker or a heckler in the crowd—what do you do?

That's what I'm going to cover right now, so I'll see you on the next page.

# Chapter 8

# Speak Up; I Can't Hear You!



## Five Characters You'll Meet on the Road

Life as an event speaker can be hilarious at times. I've had fire alarms pulled on me that evacuated the room and shut the event down in Birmingham; I've *boogie*-danced in front of a crowd in Singapore, with my team cheering and clapping me on; and I've spent 2 hours consoling a potential buyer who suffered a sad loss in the family, only to realise later that this lady was talking about her 2 cats.

She never bought in the end.

I've even had to politely escort a troublemaker to exit the conference because she was giving out a really negative vibe, disturbing the other participants, and making an overall fuss about the morning's training on day one. After she got her refund and left the building, the audience applauded; I got instant *hero* status with the room.

Life on the road is exciting, and you get to meet a lot of different characters.

I love speaking at multi-day events in front of an intimate audience of 30 to 100 people. You really get to build rapport, shift people's lives, and bring home the bacon. Over time, you'll come across some distinct characters.

I've nailed it down to 5 archetypes that you'll meet as you speak to audiences around the world.

**The Teacher**. They're the first eager-beavers to raise their hand to answer your questions, and they love to share their opinions and teach the room. They're typically highly skilled and an expert, or have had some sort of professional degree in their industry niche. But they also have a chip on their shoulder, and want the whole room to know that. They tend to attract their own little, small group entourage during breaks, and assume an unofficial leader role. You need to delicately shut them down from the get-go, as they could damage your room energy, and spread a lot of negativity among your participants. A well trained team will spot that quick, and skillfully break up any groups that might be forming. Usually, you target the leader, join the group, praise how smart they are, and then pull them aside because you have something you want to talk to them about—it works every time!.

**The Quiet Loner**. This character is going to be your biggest paying client. They're quiet, and they isolate themselves from the rest of the participants. They are the thinkers, and they are likely connecting the final dots before making that life-shifting decision. I had one client who sat in the front row to my right, and didn't open his mouth for 3 days, until we found out that he was incredibly shy and would panic every time I asked the room a question: he would just sink down into his chair and avoid any contact to being picked. He ended up investing in the highest program I was selling that weekend in Hong Kong, priced in the multiple five figures range.

***The Hugger.*** You can spot this person a mile away: They're all bubbly, touchy-feely, and appear to be in permanent happy mode. They usually come in small groups. They're a great tool for you to tap into when you need some help waking up the room, like during the post-lunch lull, or firing up some nitro-blasts of energy as you're about to introduce a new section in the training program. They have been my saving grace at times when I've had to restore the room. This character typically wants to be part of the cool crowd, but unfortunately, rarely buys.

***The Nego.*** These are your negative types. Everything to them is a scam and a lie. The internet is a scam. No one can be trusted. Usually, they've had some major setbacks in their life, and brought that *baggage* with them into the room. The full onslaught of negativity rears its ugly head, typically, toward the back end of your event. They start complaining that there's too much selling and not enough teaching, and that the room is too hot or too cold. The Wi-Fi sucks, somebody stinks, their favorite cookies weren't available at the coffee breaks, and why isn't lunch included...whatever!! As the speaker and CEO of the room, you have to respectfully agree, and defer to your team to handle their issues during the break. I've had to refund many tickets in the past. It's best to nip negativity in the bud, before it contaminates the room and wipes out your, and your team's, pay check at the end of the event.

***The Marty McFly.*** Remember the movie, *Back to the Future?* "Hello...McFly...hello...hello?" The lights are on but nobody's home. This character is stuck in oblivion, and they would answer *yes* to literally every question you ask them, but they really have no clue what the question is about. They are your walking zombies, taking up dead space in the room. They flow in and out of your event, and you never knew who they were.

You're always going to get these characters in your room. That's why it's so important to work with your team on day 1, to figure out who's in the room: where your hot buyers are; and your marginals (people who can be pulled into as buyers but are sitting on the fence). It directs your focus and sales energy for day two, on pitching and selling, and closing and collecting the money on day three.

## HOW to Open Your Mouth and Get Paid Thousands of Dollars...PER HOUR

There's never a direct way to becoming a speaker and landing gigs that pay you thousands of dollars per hour. But first things first: You must be trained in the art of speaking and selling.

You need to invest in a coach or mentor, or preferably someone who has active speaking engagements, who may not give you a lot of time or attention due to their hectic schedule on the road. Ideally, the mentor who really has the time to guide you on your way to speaking from the stage, is ideally somebody who knows how to teach speaking and selling from the stage, through a system, and who has had a lot of experience in the profession.

Speaking and getting paid has nothing to do with getting up in front of an audience and talking about what you know. There are a series of skills that take into account your choice of words, the psychology of the room, storytelling, conscious and subconscious communication, embedded commands, and all the tiny nuances that happen every minute you're on stage, which ultimately moves the audience one step closer to rushing to the back of the room, with credit card in hand.

Another consideration in evaluating a coach or mentor, or somebody to train you, is to what extent they have access to a network of events and organisers that can help plan your first speaking gig, so that you can start getting noticed by the world.

If you ever land your first gig, or get a chance to speak for free in front of a live audience, get it filmed...even if it's your friend with your smartphone. The video and pictures of you speaking in front of an audience will instantly brand you as a credible speaker, and leverage your digital assets in your marketing.

My son's a filmmaker. When I brought him to the UK, I decided to try and get his first gig as a commercial videographer in the event seminar space. He ended up travelling around the world for a year, filming, and surrounding himself with some pretty successful people. We've even done events together, which has been just amazing, and I obviously leverage those fringe benefits: He has filmed and photographed me, and I've used those video clips to get noticed for other speaking engagements.

My wife and I are both trained and professional international speakers. We normally take on board a few special clients at a time, due to the personal nature and time-commitment required to train and adapt to our clients' needs. It has to be a right fit for both client and us. One major way to qualify our clients for this special speaker training relationship is by using The BrandQ Methodology™ and The BrandQ Value Ladder Blueprint™. It is with this process that we can objectively assess and help the client truly see whether speaking on a stage is essential to their branding and positioning, or whether it would be just nice to have. They also must be coachable. The relationship doesn't work if the new client already has an idea of what speaking is all about. If it's a fit, then it's an amazing journey that we're both on.

Your local Toastmasters chapter is a really good way to consistently get the opportunity to speak in front of a crowd every other week. Much of the time, it's impromptu speaking to sharpen your craft, and it's a lot of fun. Keep in mind that this kind of speaking is usually more about getting the applause of appreciation, and less about learning how to command a room to part with their money.

## WHERE to Open Your Mouth and Get Paid Thousands of Dollars…PER HOUR

There are several different formats of speaking gigs, and I'll give you an idea behind the structure of the deal so that you can figure out where you see yourself, and how much you want to earn as a speaker.

Regardless of the event format, your expenses for getting to and from the event are covered by the host organiser: air tickets (normally economy class, unless you're a frequent flyer and earn your own upgrades), ground transportation, and your accommodation. Make sure the event organisers pay for the bills, rather than you paying for them first and then having to submit an expense claim. It makes sense on your cash flow.

*Free preview events:* The public attends a free event to get a 90-minute preview of a given topic, and are invited to purchase an upsell to a follow-up program or workshop. This is a very different speaking style that is high energy and just enough content to raise the audience's curiosity to want more. Your speaking structure will be geared toward making a minimum of 3 sales pitches: in the first 10 minutes of speaking; then at the 45-minute mark; and then at the 60-minute mark (usually done a few times using different room closing techniques), to send buyers to the back of the room to purchase a ticket for a multi-day workshop, with bonuses, priced anywhere between $400 to $700.

Your contract deal is anywhere from 10% to 20% of the gross revenue sales of every ticket sold at the event when you're the speaker (sometimes you'll split sessions with another speaker, but it's unusual). Your target conversion rate to shoot for is a minimum of 20%. When you can convert a *cold room* at this rate (a room full of strangers who don't know who you are or the product you're selling), you're solid and reliable enough to have the company or organiser invite you back. The higher your conversion rate, the higher chance that you're put on a longer contract. Free event formats usually spread over 2 to 3 days, with two to three 90-minute sessions a day. So it can be very exhausting, even though the sessions are short. Depending on the product pricing, room size, your conversion rate, and the number of sessions you're speaking at, you could be taking home several thousand or upwards of $10,000 for 2 to 3 days of speaking. Do a couple of these a month regularly, and you're on your way to becoming a millionaire speaker!

***Pitch-fests or multi-speaker events:*** These are events where you are one of several speakers pitching your $1,000 to $3,000 product on stage for 90 minutes. Audience sizes at these events can be several thousand people. This is a unique format in which all the revenue you sell is yours (if it's your own product), but you have to split the share, sometimes up to 50%, with the organiser, for bringing the event and audience together. Consider it a distribution fee. Typically, the speaker is the one who created their own product and is doing the selling, so he or she keeps all the revenue from sales, and splits the proceeds with the event organiser.

***Multi-day workshop seminars:*** One of the highest paid speaker roles is when you are hired as the lead trainer and speaker (i.e. the only speaker) for a multi-day event. A separate deal structure is usually negotiated, which includes expenses and accommodation, plus anywhere up to 15% of the total revenue collected by the end of that event, and a slightly reduced percentage of the remaining fees that will be collected over the next 30 to 45 days after the event. Don't worry about this, as it will be your sales team following up with clients on collecting the payment balances from deposits paid at the event.

The amount you can expect to earn from a multi-day event will really depend on the types of products and services being offered by the company you're speaking for, and the price points...and obviously, how well you close. The business coaching and consultation niche programs typically range from several thousand dollars all the way up to tens of thousands of dollars, and even over a hundred thousand dollars (yes, you need training on how to sell a $100,000 program). I was lead speaker and trainer for several different companies, both on the free and multi-day event formats. I would be doing two free event series, plus one to two multi-day events per month. Let's just say that I would take home more money from a weekend event than I was earning in a month when I was still in a corporate job.

The free, plus 3-day, event format series is a very popular speaker event, structured for companies in the event seminar niche.

***The Mastermind Event:*** I love these events that usually take place at an exotic, 5-star resort location. It's a small event format, with an audience size of up to 50 clients who have paid a lot of money to be there to be trained. This is your *warm audience,* as they are existing clients who have bought multiple times and have clearly benefited and want more specialized training. This is called a mastermind format event. Your focus, as a lead speaker, trainer, and host, is less of the hard-selling characteristic of the other event formats. It's much more about relationship-selling, and really getting into the problem-solving aspect of your client, and offering tailored solutions.

Your speaker compensation ranges between 4 to 6% of sales from the event. This is because the hard work has already been done with getting a cold audience to buy. Normally, companies may offer to compensate you for this lower commission, by way of a flat fee you receive just for getting on a plane. In any case, you have the luxury of staying and working in exotic locations, and it's a great branding piece for your brand. So, you need to look at the total package and not just the commission piece.

I have extensive experience with all three formats, on a regular monthly basis, and I can tell you that the amount of branding this has done for me has been immeasurable.

Imagine the reaction you get when you tell people you're a speaker—Wow!!

And then, when you tell them you're an international speaker—Wow, wow!!

Or, if you tell them you're a lead trainer for multi-day workshops—Whoop, whoop!!

And you're a speaker and a mentor to elite VIP clientele at five star resort mastermind events— WOOOOWWWW!!

Now, that's the tip of the iceberg…

Learning how to speak and sell is not only reserved for being on a stage in front of a live audience. This skill has another important application...and that is speaking to sell on a webinar.

When you can command an audience with storytelling, value, and connecting the dots in your online audience's mind, your sales closing techniques are going to be very similar to closing clients on a live webinar behind your $500, $1000, $2000, or $3000 product.

Get the webinar right, record it, and set it in an automated webinar funnel, and your recorded speech will make you money without you even putting on your best suit.

Now, do you see how the skill of speaking is so powerful?

## Twelve Survival Tips to Speaking on the Road

So, are you ready to become a speaker now? Are you committed to getting trained? Is speaking-to-many congruent with your brand, and the absolute best platform to blast your message out to the world?

Money and power makes you more of the person you are already. It will change you either positively or negatively. And that will depend on you.

I tend to discourage people from making the jump into speaking unless I sense they have their head screwed on right. There is a *rock-star* feeling that comes with the territory: the spotlight, the money, the attention. If you're not properly grounded, you'll fall into the usual traps of drugs, alcohol, or sex, which has destroyed lives and families.

It is a serious business, from a material, emotional, and spiritual standpoint, in becoming a speaker.

So as not to end this chapter on a down note, how about I leave you with my 12 survival tips guide to the road of speaking.

#1: Travel in comfort (and I'm not talking first-class, as chances are, your hiring company or event organizer is not going to be covering this class of travel). Definitely enroll in all your airline frequent flyer programs if this is going to be a regular thing, and try to fly on those airlines as much as you can, to rack up the miles for your next first-class upgrade. Take as direct a flight as possible, and minimize the number of stops. Arrive a day early to decompress (especially if you're travelling across multiple time zones), and leave 1 day after you have finished. It pays dividends to leave the event the following day so that you have an evening to treat your team to dinner.

#2: De-stress when you arrive. I love speaking in Asia, especially in Thailand, as I get to go to my favourite massage place for a facial, foot shiatsu, and traditional Thai massage. Head to the hotel sauna or gym to sweat out the travel aches and lethargy. You need to be in tip-top shape for the next few days.

#3: Pack your suits in a bag to avoid wrinkling. In addition to your suit cover, I find that it helps to layer it with sheets of plastic bags. If you need a final touch up on your outfit, proceed to the next tip.

#4: Learn how to iron, and definitely pack a small can of spray starch. Most often, your hiring event organiser or agent will not cover room incidentals like laundry or the mini bar. Even if you pay for it yourself, you can never guarantee that housekeeping will get it done when you want it. Always control the variables so that you are in your comfort zone with your immediate environment.

#5: Invest in a good sound system, and take it with you...everywhere. I never ever use supplied equipment. I need to have confidence in my equipment's quality, so I take and use my own. It's like underwear. Never use someone else's!! And that includes your own computer, cable connections, adaptors, and clicker. You never want to rely on crappy hotel equipment, because it's unreliable, especially since, over the years, hotels have subcontracted out to third party suppliers. Most often, the sound system speakers are fine, but if you're going to take speaking seriously, invest in a top of the line, wireless microphone that you hang around your head—the protective case that it comes with will fit snugly in your suitcase. The quality of your overall delivery has a direct link to your paycheck and family's livelihood, so it pays to invest wisely in your craft.

#6: Get the energy flowing at the start of the morning. Go for a run, work out, meditate, pray, psych yourself up in the mirror...whatever suits your fancy. You want to be energized the moment you head downstairs and it's *game time*. Always remember to take deep steady breaths, to get oxygen flowing in your bloodstream.

#7: Leave your *crap* out of the room...and that goes for your team members too. There is absolutely no room for negativity, from you or your team, to enter the room: something happened at home, or you got into an argument, or you're going through a divorce...whatever; never bring that into the room—because the energy you carry is the energy you create, which transmits to your audience.

#8: Absolutely no alcohol during the event. I make it a point to avoid any alcohol, because it makes me tired. Some speakers have a night-cap to ease the nerves, so there's no hard and fast rules. The point is that you need a good night's rest. It's exhilarating and exhausting as a speaker. Most of the fatigue comes from the adrenaline pumping through your veins the entire day. Do the necessary debriefings with your team on the day's results and game plan for the next day, and then head straight to your room. After the event is over, it's always great to throw back a few and just decompress with your team — especially if you work with them quite frequently. The unwritten rule is to treat your team well, and get the Starbucks coffee in the morning, and host a casual dinner on the last night. They will bend over backwards for you for future events...and you'll need all the support in the room you can get.

#9: Dress for your *A-Game*. You must feel successful. As far as you're concerned, you're the *guru* in the room. Don't overdo it with flash; you'll come across as being a bit too much *into yourself*, and usually, when speakers are self-absorbed, the audience perceives it as being all about you, and not them, as it should be. On a 3-day workshop event, I'm usually in a light blue shirt and dark suit on day one, as it's neutral; then I switch to a grey shirt and light pink shirt for day-2's product pitch day. Pink is a secret color that tells the audience, "Hey, it's safe." Then, on day 3, when I'm focused on closing-training-closing, I'm more relaxed in a black t-shirt with a grey blazer and black jeans, and then I pull out my secret weapon: my *Christian Louboutin*, python skin, chrome-studded loafers!! This really gets the crowd going because, I know, every time, I've built a very good rapport with the audience...and I like to have a bit of fun and leave the audience on a high note, so that if they don't buy that weekend, they'll buy next time!!

#10: Protect and conserve your voice. You want to limit your speaking to the stage, and avoid lengthy discussions and chatter between days. Also, pace yourself throughout the event. You don't want to over-exert your energy and strain your voice, and struggle on the back end of the event, especially if your voice starts crackling and you're feeling energy-sapped at the time of pitching and closing—your most important part because that's about the money. It's like a 15-round fight: You need to be able to go the distance. I always used to get reminded to breathe and slow down, by my on-site mentor, who was also my director of events. It's good to have a coach on your team, to observe and give you feedback when you need to hear it. Of course, on shorter, 90-minute events, go all out!!!

#11: Eat light during the event. You don't want to have indigestion, having to taste that delicious *tandoori* curry chicken bubbling up in your throat!  Remember, you have a lip microphone right by your mouth, so any sound that emerges (like burping) will sound like a freakin' fog horn in the room.

#12: Always have good breath. There's nothing worse than sitting in the front row with the stench coming from the speaker's mouth, smelling like he ate a dead cat for breakfast. Chew sugarless gum (sugar creates bacteria in your mouth), and brush your teeth and tongue during the day at breaks. Avoid coffee, as it dries your mouth, and you'll start making those annoying *chapping* sounds in your mic as your lips and tongue smack against the dry walls of your mouth. When this happens, you also tend to hurl spit projectiles into the front row—trust me, I've had embarrassing and hilarious moments on the road. One lady, in Hong Kong, opened up an umbrella, inside the room, while I was speaking!  The joke was well taken and really got the participants going. You need to have a healthy sense of humour about yourself, and not take yourself too seriously. Self-deprecation makes you human, and your audience will love you.

And a BONUS for you, lucky #13: Reaffirm why you're on the road, because it can get lonely. I always have an open bible set up on my table, with a verse that means a lot to me, along with pictures of my wife and kids. I saw a renowned speaker doing this one time, and I asked them about it. "It reminds me of my *'why,'*" they said.

I liked that, and so it stuck.

I'm going to switch gears in the next chapter, because it's an important one for you. You may have the perfect brand, the perfect product, the perfect funnel, the perfect marketing, and you're a world-class speaker. But still, something's missing. You're stuck, and you're wondering, "What's going on?"

Why is success so elusive? Why are you still not achieving the results you want, despite doing all the right things?

The next chapter may provide you the deeper answers to the questions you have.

See you in a few.

# Chapter 9

# The Turning Point with Haggai

*"…and I will make you like a signet ring, for I have chosen you,
says the Lord of Hosts."*
– The Book of Haggai (Old Testament NKJV)

## Is Your Business Grounded Correctly?

We moved back to Hong Kong, in 2013, after I lost my job, and we lived 3 years out of a typically tiny apartment on the Southside of Hong Kong Island. My wife and I started a business in organic acai (pronounced *asai*) fruit juices.

Susy and I knew we had a winner on our hands.

We weren't prepared to put a lot of money in this fledgling business to plough into warehousing and storage costs. By the way, if you've never been to Hong Kong, it's extremely dense and over-populated. Space is a premium, and very, very, very expensive. Rent is a killer. We live in match boxes stacked 90 floors high! Fun fact: The average Hong Konger lives 17 floors above ground, the highest altitude urban population in the world.

125

We used our small living room to store the half pallet of fruit juices, and dropped orders to our restaurant customers.

Then, one day, I was working out of a cafe in the city when I got an urgent call from the building management of our apartment complex. They asked me to come home immediately.

There was water gushing out of our apartment—say whaaaaat??!!

My heart raced into panic mode as I grabbed the next taxi and rushed home. As I entered the apartment building lobby, water was dripping into the elevator shaft, and it had short-circuited the elevator of the twenty-three floor building. I raced up fourteen flights of stairs, to our 7th floor home, and faced the horror. The hallway was flooded, and water was pouring out from under our apartment door. I fumbled around for my keys, tears welling up in my eyes as I opened the door.

There was over an inch of water in my living room. The kitchen was a complete wreck, with water and debris all over the place. It looked as if a bomb had gone off!

Construction workers, who were renovating the apartment directly above us, broke a water main pipe, which flooded upstairs, and to make matters worse, the negligent workers punctured a pipe that led down into our apartment unit. All the water and crap from upstairs flowed straight into our home.

Our sanctuary was a disaster zone.

I immediately called Susy. You can only imagine the shock on her face when she saw the state of our apartment. After half an hour of screaming and threats of lawsuits, the cleanup crew from the complex came in to vacuum all the excess surface water. The landlord from upstairs emerged with his contractors, and assured us everything would be taken care of. No worries!

So, we began itemizing every piece of damage that needed replacing. My heart sank when our beautiful Turkish carpet, which I had spent hours haggling over, near the Blue Mosque in Istanbul, was completely damaged.

The biggest heartbreak was that all our remaining acai fruit juice cartons were contaminated from the water and debris. There was no way we could sell them, and we wrote off the entire stock that had literally washed away.

A slow legal process ensued. A year passed, and the judge finally found no fault on the upstairs landlord for negligence. Due to a technicality, responsibility fell on the contractors. But they disappeared. Their business license and registration expired 2 years ago, and technically, there was no way to pursue the case.

We got screwed by an unforgiving system. And that was the end of our first venture.

What happened? Why did this happen to us? Why? Why? Why?

My network marketing business really didn't take off either. I did all the training. I met with people. People didn't show up to coffee meetings. I recruited downlines who gave up. In 18 months, I was going nowhere with this business.

You know the feeling you get when you're doing all the work, you follow the process, you grind away, and nothing happens? Is it me?

You may have a terrific product. You may have great marketing, your mindset is good, and you have trusted staff—and still your business can tank before it even gets off the ground.

I consider myself to be a relatively intelligent guy who can figure things out, having over 20 years business experience...why couldn't I make my own business work for me? I saw other successful people all around me. Why?

Fast forward a few years, and I was growing two burgeoning online marketing businesses. At one stage, I had four streams of cash flow from multiple businesses. Life was finally taking a turn for the better, and the grind was starting to pay off. We even moved to the UK for a much better quality of life.

But all that came crashing down. Again.

You know, it's funny. When things are going well, you appreciate the tough times of the past and the life challenges that prepare you for the person you are becoming. You're full of gratitude, and everything smells rosy. Then life has a sense of humour. It wants to test you again. It says, *"Well, if you made it through that, try this on for size."*

Successful business owners are often asked whether they would do it over again, knowing what they know today in achieving their success. The typical answer is "of course"—it's the journey.

I call *BS*! No one ever wants to start over.

My wife and I have been through some tough times: battling cancer, being laid off, being unemployable at forty-three, having a flooded home, and starting and closing several businesses.

Okay, we get it! What does life have to teach us this time? So many questions; no answers.

I was broken.

Little did I know that a couple months after my consultancy business took a major setback, I would begin to truly understand why I was taken out of that business. It was guidance. It was a message. And I understood why.

It absolutely crushed and humbled me. But there was a deeper lesson to take in.

My business wasn't grounded properly.

## A World Littered by Paradox

Six months prior to all this turmoil, I renewed my walk with the Lord after 20 years of neglecting Him. Yeah, I was still chasing the wrong things. Everything I had done to date was through what I believed was my own doing—the work of my own hands, my intellect, my own ability on my terms. I didn't ask any permission from the Great Counsellor. I did not seek His advice in pretty much everything I did. We spoke on and off for over 20 years. Like a child leaving his father to venture out into the world alone: *Leave me alone Dad; I'll call when I can...I got this!!*

My life and businesses were grounded in sand that were swept away by the tempestuous winds of change.

I misappropriated my funds without advice, and racked up huge credit card debt. I got into businesses for the money. I was chasing an empty dream that could never be fulfilled. I was heading to eventual self destruction and a life of emptiness, without even knowing. My purpose was noble: serving and educating people around the world, and providing for my family. But I wanted to do it on my terms. I was self-serving. I was seeking my own god, and the one true God was giving me a nudge and a serious wake up call.

I hate religion. I despise church hypocrisy, and I've got a pretty sensitive BS meter when it comes to religious figures. I gave my life to the Lord, at a big outreach when I was 17, and I walked and preached my faith throughout my college years. But greed in making money, and creating something of my own life, took over. All these years, I knew I was being watched over, but I brushed those voices aside, saying, "I'll get back to you later. It's my time now."

I came across the book of Haggai, in the Old Testament. It hit me like a sledgehammer. It's a great book on business for any entrepreneur. It's a revelation you must understand behind the pursuit of what you want in life. There is also a deeper meaning inside, which teaches you how to ground your life goals and business correctly.

We've put our Creator aside.

The world has made significant advances in technology, and we've been able to harness the power of medicine to extend life and cure disease. We have the capacity to produce enough food to feed the world many times over, and to erect engineering miracles that define our imagination; and we have the brilliance to send man and machine to explore the far edges of the universe.

You have, in essence, put the power of God into your own hands, in the *rat race* pursuit of defining your life meaning, fooling yourself that you don't need God, and yet you are not filled with God.

Our world is crumbling.

Despite advances in medical technology and human capability, we experience widespread famine, with many living without food each day, nor having access to clean water or basic health care. Big governments lend money to poor nations, and hold the debt ransom in exchange for exclusive resource rights, fattening the coffers of big corporations, and widening the gap between the *haves* and the *have-nots*.

Social values are collapsing despite medical advances to heal the weak. We create new diseases in the fabric of society, and threaten to annihilate each other with weapons of mass destruction, all in the name of peace.

We live in a world of paradoxes.

We have completely lost sight of Him, yet we seek our own immortality through our own works. We seek God in other forms—idols, New Age thinking, and introducing rituals into our lives to make us feel spiritual—yet we are not full of the Spirit. We celebrate creation but not the Creator.

Instead of rooting ourselves back to where we came from, we procrastinate and press the pause button; we create new ideas and confuse ourselves into feeling an alternative sense of godliness.

We fool ourselves with being in control, but we are not. And life has a way of reminding us of our own mortality.

We preach spirituality and godly ways; we dive into avenues of idolatry and beliefs, yet we're prepared to kill each other because of our values, differences in our backgrounds, and the color of our skin.

We look for new lands because mankind has outgrown its home, reaching out into deep space for salvation.

The Earth is sick. And so are we.

## Why You Are Not Profiting in the Marketplace...Yet

We are destroying God's house and have left His temple in ruins. And that includes surrendering our spirit and body into slavery. You're likely imprisoned in a job you already hate and dread. Someone else has taken your time away, but in return has taken your worth for granted by not paying you what you truly deserve.

We continue to demonstrate the unbelievable feats of what mankind is capable of in the fields of science and technology. Examples abound in our ability to overcome challenges and show compassion. Miracles are around us, and yet we are blinded by our own lack of belief and cynicism; and while we have a capacity for greatness, we also have the ability for doing unthinkable evil.

You know how to live materially, but your life lacks fulfillment.

Countless stories abound with the materially wealthy, yet they live in the anguish of drugs,
addiction, failed marriages, sickness, and loneliness, and their children don't want anything to do with them.

One of the most heart crushing realities of this fact is about a man who had an abundance of wealth, fame, and fortune, and a global following of admirers...he made the world laugh, yet he was in deep depression.

A man of great wit and humor and ended up threading a noose around his head, hanging himself naked in his own bathroom.

His name, was Robin Williams.

*"Is it time for you yourselves to dwell in your panelled houses,*
*and this temple to lie in ruins?"*
*You have sown much, and bring in little;*
*You eat, but do not have enough;*
*You drink, but you are not filled with drink;*
*You dothe yourselves, but no one is warm;*
*And he who earns wages,*
*Earns wages to put into a bag with holes."*
(Haggai 1:4-6)

I lived 22 years plundering after my desires ...pursuing a dream that was not mine. I was living an ideal that was created by society for me. I did the school thing, and I did it well. I pursued the job career, made vast sums of money for somebody else, and was handsomely rewarded as a result.

I built and lived in my own panelled house...and neglected His temple.

Mistakes started manifesting themselves into my life, the price of which I've paid for...

But the debt is now settled by the grace of the Lord, through the Blood of Christ. Yet His temple remains in ruins...and He is calling us to take care of it first, before the gifts from above can truly manifest themselves in our lives.

It's a cool, misty night on a hilltop residential community in São Paulo, Brazil. For the second time in five years, I'm an invited guest in the home of an individual who has amassed a fortune in his lifetime as an inventor.

He's an avid tennis player, as am I. It's a rematch of five years prior...Game on! But this time, I see a different opponent. Something about him has changed. There's a humility I see now that I didn't see back 5 years ago when we first met.

After the game, we head back to his condo to freshen up, and I sink into his plush sofa in the middle of his sprawling pad.

Material riches and symbols of his wealth are everywhere. His lovely wife cooks us a well- deserved meal, a piping hot, local delicacy. His 11-year-old son is glued to me with admiration, basking in the rare presence of a *foreign* house guest, who is speaking Portuguese with a funny accent.

My host turns to me and asks what's happened in my life since our last meeting. I go on to explain the years of struggle, having lost my job after a 22-year career, my wife's battle with cancer, and the death of my father.

He ponders what I tell him, like a wise sage. It was his turn.

He recounts his story of how a rare blood disease almost took his life a couple of years ago. As he speaks, his eyes well up in tears. But those are not tears of sadness or remorse... *"They are tiny streams of happiness, joy, and rebirth,"* he explains.

He looks up from gazing down at the floor, and tells me, "Ian...I had to face what my life had amounted to. Emptiness."

He had it all; all the material wealth and comfort one can only dream of.

He continues, "There is a time in your life, Ian, when you have to take a lesson from Him...on your knees."

The Lord sent me a message.

Six months later, I rededicated my life to Him. I was reborn again, my debt repaid... in the Blood of Christ and the Holy Spirit.

For so many years, I pursued money and thought I was doing well. Then it all came crashing down like the proverbial house of cards.

It was time to rebuild—this time with a house built on bedrock.

## Loading up the Storehouses

Cynical, angry, and skeptical of the world, I was disillusioned with the world of entrepreneurship. I knew it would be hard, and I put in the grind and invested in myself, but finding the success I desired was elusive.

*"You looked for much, but indeed it came to little; and when you brought it home, I blew it away. Why?" says the Lord of Hosts. "Because of My house that is in ruins, while every one of you withhold the dew, and the earth withholds the fruit. For I called for a drought on the land and the mountains, on the grain and the new wine and the oil, on whatever the ground brings forth, on men and livestock, and on all the labor of your hands."*
(Haggai 1:9-11)

It seemed like every time I built a business, it was all taken away…in an instant. Such is the cruelty of business—and of life, and of thinking of myself before our Maker.

The Lord's temple must come first before anything else. The temple is not a physical structure but a temple that resides in you.

The Lord resides in me. He resides in you, whether you know Him or not.

It requires housecleaning, putting a new order and structure so that He may be glorified. All the things we pursue in this life… fulfilment, purpose, material wealth, possessions, peace, and all the clichés that industry and self-help gurus teach, and that we have been conditioned into wanting by mass media and social expectations…these all belong to Him. *"The silver is Mine, and the gold is Mine."* (Haggai 2:8)

The struggles and challenges we face in the pursuit of that which we choose to attain, is not without walking the fine line of duality: the truth that keeps us on this path, and the opposites of truth that aim to dislodge us.

It does require that we load up the storehouses. What this means is to show our gratitude for the success and the results we achieve in our life, by giving back. It's like energy. For more to come in, more must flow out, so that we become renewed and ready to receive more. The more output we give, the more input we receive.

Tithing and offering has its roots in the Bible, but the modern TV evangelist and head of the local church has perverted its deeper spiritual meaning. It is no wonder why we cringe when the subject of tithes and offerings is brought up. But the spiritual meaning is a return and multiplication of what we gladly give.

2 Corinthians 9:6–15 talks about being a cheerful giver; giving with your heart, expecting nothing in return. God wants you to

live in prosperity, so He wants to give back tenfold what you offer. If you knew you could receive ten times what you offer, wouldn't everyone be doing that...especially in our age of *WIIFM* (what's-in-it-for-me)? Our own prejudices keep us from doing it, as we have turned our backs on man's religion. But we shouldn't turn our backs to God.

It does say, in Malachi 3:8–12, that we can test God on his word by giving: *"Bring all the tithes into the storehouse, that there may be food in My house, and try Me now in this," says the Lord of hosts. "If I will not open for you the windows of heaven and pour out for you such blessing that there will not be room enough to receive it."*

Whenever I receive a new increase, new customers, or a major new client, these are called *First Fruits*. I know that if I offer it all back, more will come. Proverbs 3:9–10 says, *"Honor the Lord with your possessions, and with the first fruits of all your increase; so your barns will be filled with plenty, and your vats will overflow with new wine."*

## Living in Abundance

Only with Him, in Him, and through Him can you enjoy the abundance that is promised to you in this life and eternally. All these things must be purified and in alignment to allow the abundance of the Lord to flow through.

And you can count on his promise...by His grace that led the children of Israel out of Egypt, the Lord Almighty made a covenant to protect his people...and so shall He protect you. And you should not fear (Haggai 2:5).

The temple that is within you must be purified in all senses: ridding the garments of idolatry, of ego; cutting off the curses that have subdued your potential, and that which have been the cables from the generational garments and misfortune that have cloaked you; to now dedicating all that you do in life to Him, honouring Him in spirit. The thoughts that enter your mind, how you respond to them, and becoming conscious of what comes out of your mouth can be either a blessing or a curse.

In the early chapters, I taught you that one of the biggest moves to survive and make it in the entrepreneur world is a complete change of self. Your old habits and belief systems got you to where you are…and are unlikely to take you further, especially if you know you need to make that big shift. Your old self has to "die," and you have to start feeding in new stimulus to create a version of you that is going to succeed as a business owner, creating your own economy.

You literally have to be a completely new person…and I'm not talking about character or personality here. I'm talking about a complete new operating software system that powers your brain, your emotions, and physical being.

I told you about my 20-year addiction to cigarettes. Yes, I can finally admit it now. I was addicted, and I was in denial, kidding myself that I could quit anytime.

I knew I wanted to get healthy. I was into cycling. I had my nemesis of a hill climb that I wanted to conquer. But I could only get through the climb if I cleaned myself up. And I did.

I realised, to get what you want in life, you need to look at the benefits and rewards. Otherwise, a goal is absent, and has no bearing and context. I finally attached a resulting benefit that I could feel from quitting smoking: being able to do a hill climb at a 15% gradient. Your body is a temple that needs cleaning up. Reboot the mind, clean up the body, and eliminate all the bad habits.

And that's just the beginning of a lifelong journey. You will slip—and that's expected—and it's OK.

I wake up each morning and ask Him: "Good morning...what's Your plan today...what are we to achieve together today?" People set aside their own quiet time, or prayer time, or whatever you want to call it, to center themselves for the day. Do you do that? I encourage you to do so. And if you find you're in a better place, try doing it throughout the day. Give thanks, and ask questions....your downloads will come, and your instincts and intuition (I call it moving in the Spirit) will lead you to the right decisions. There have been countless occasions where my old self would try to dictate that I make the wrong money decisions, and so many times, I have been pulled away from making them.

More recently, I was attending a guru workshop, and there was a very high level training being offered to attend an exclusive $10,000 mindset training that could fix how to manifest what we want in life...guaranteed. My wife, Susy, and I were really tempted but had a few questions for the guru before pulling out our credit cards.

Thank God, this guru was swamped by workshop participants, and we couldn't get to him. I took a moment, paused, and ask the Great Counsellor for some guidance. We then decided to leave the room for a while, away from the hype, to take a restroom break. Later that afternoon, in plain view, we could discern with a sharper vision, the guru's values and true intentions. We just didn't feel right about making that kind of investment in him. Although the subject matter was intriguing and important for our education journey as entrepreneurs, Susy and I decided not to choose this particular guru to be our teacher...and we walked away $10,000 richer in our pockets.

I got the message.

## The Chairman of Your Board

There is nothing more reassuring than the deep faith and knowing that the Man upstairs has got your back.

I grew up without going to church. My father, Nico, who was a Roman Catholic, had very strong Christian values instilled in him by his parents. Fighting between the Catholics and Protestants in Northern Ireland caused my grandfather to leave the church of hypocrisy. Nico was a heavy smoker. He had many Christian friends, and one of them, a fellow Roman Catholic, was so devout in his faith, forcing his beliefs on his fellow heathens, that he would often ridicule my dad into not having the strength or willpower to be able to quit his nasty habit. With a gentlemanly pride, he gracefully told the guy, "*Up yours,*" and never smoked again after that life-altering day.

Naysayers can inadvertently become our greatest motivators in life.

It irritates the heck out of me how church-going Christians, who appear to do all the right things in everyone's eyes, flaunt their piousness onto others. And on the other hand, I think it's really *off* when you see a lot of other Christians taking such a passive stance on life, praying and leaving everything in God's hands, then sitting back, waiting, and saying, "If it's God's will."

God does not teach us to become passive Christians. He charges us with spreading the word of salvation. He teaches us how to deal with the enemy. He shows us how to arm ourselves when we proactively go into battle in the marketplace. He teaches us how to listen with a discerning ear, on when to make decisions and how to separate opportunity from threat. He shields his soldiers charged to make a difference in the marketplace, in ministry, with our families, in our community, in service, and in the products and services we create as entrepreneurs, to solve the world's problems.

You are the chief executive officer of your business. You are charged with the executive powers to implement strategies, exploit growth opportunities, and build an organisation of leaders who will grow your company's influence and impact with your clients and consumers.

But like all CEOs of major corporations, there is the *big boss*: the *chairman of the board*.

A chairman, by definition, is an executive elected by the company's board of directors. He oversees the board's mandate to establish policies for corporate management, governance, and oversight, and has a major sway in the decision-making process on major company issues. He takes into account the interests of both internal and external stakeholders of a company. The chairman does not undermine the responsibility of the CEO, but rather serves as the CEO's mentor, advisor, and confidante in the smooth running of the company, in ensuring performance excellence in the marketplace.

Rooting your company's purpose in God, and appointing Him as chairman of the board, is a powerful reassurance that you'll be able to guide your business spiritually and physically so that He may be praised, and in return, He will make you like the signet ring of association in Him, marked by His seal. He will bless your business, your products and services, your profits, your employees, and your legal environment, and guide you through the guarantee of challenge, as you gather the marketplace around you for His glory.

A signet ring is a symbol of heritage, marked by a seal, which indicates an affiliation. It is a ring that will be bestowed upon you. You must always honor it, respect it, and give glory to the One you received it from, never taking it for granted, nor let your ego rule over it. *"...and I will make you like a signet ring, for I have chosen you, says the Lord of Hosts."* (Haggai 2:22)

And so, the ultimate question for your business is this: What is your purpose in serving Him?

That was the question I pondered after I read the Book of Haggai. I've heard it said that once your mission and vision are crystal clear of what you want to achieve through your business, the rest just takes care of itself.

Having been lost and confused with my own clarity, I did receive these spiritual downloads (or messages) after studying the Book of Haggai:

I am in the business of helping people create freedom for themselves.

I am in the business of freeing people from the shackles of poverty and enslavement to a broken system…and to a wrong master.

I am in the business of prosperity and wealth in creating independent and free living.

I am in the business of creating sustainable livelihoods and family.

I am in the business of independent learning and education and knowledge and richness, and living life to the fullest.

I am in the business of helping people seek God through freeing them from the shackles of poverty, inspiring them through education to seek prosperity in becoming independently minded through entrepreneurship in the new economy.

I am in the business of attracting and teaching a way of hope so that through my business vehicle, more individuals can be drawn into a life of abundance and the Glory of God.

When I wrote down these downloads some time ago, I started writing the preface to this book. And I already had a name for the book title.

*The Big Shift.*

My journey of discovering myself in Him continues...

# Chapter 10

# So Where Do You Go from Here?

*"You can't help but... with 20/20 hindsight, go back and say,
'Look, had we done something different, we probably wouldn't
be facing what we are facing today.'"*
– Norman Schwarzkopf

## The Dangers of Relying on One

One of the hidden truths in the modern age is not only about being an entrepreneur and building your own economy, but also about creating multiple streams of income.

You don't want to be let go from a job and lose your only source of income, to then move into a business and depend on only one source of revenue, like in a restaurant or a consulting gig, where you're a one-trick pony. That, too, can disappear overnight from competition, reputational damage, or a failed health inspection on your premises; or your landlord decides to increase the rent of your business, or there is an increase in the cost of goods, but you've had to drop pricing to remain in business, and you're not making payroll—and your business ends up filing for bankruptcy.

Having multiple streams of income is the way forward in the new economy.

You're probably thinking, "Hang on a second, Ian. Haven't you been teaching us to start a business? And now you're saying we have to start multiple businesses? Isn't one hard enough?"

Yes, I am advising you to start multiple businesses...but doing it by leveraging the same skill set.

In the chapter on funnels, I taught you that you're going to need multiple funnels to attract different types of clientele into your business, to increase the chances of acquiring a steady flow of clients and customers; so too will you need different streams of cash flow just in case one of them fails.

At one stage, I had 5 streams of cash flow. Two of them disappeared overnight because I decided to end the contract to focus on the others. The 3 skill sets that united all these businesses together were:  communication, speaking, and marketing.

I was an affiliate marketer, promoting a company's products, and I used my knowledge to become their lead speaker and trainer. So, essentially, I expanded my income channels with just these skill sets.

There are businesses and systems for you to learn how to start your business by understanding how their systems work. Remember how I taught you that one of the core foundations of your business is to develop a turn-key operation?

Ultimately, you want to learn from other companies, with the end goal of building your own. It only takes a company to shut down; and overnight, you're out of business.

My key learning, from an episode I experienced, is to build something you own; and leverage your expertise and skills to build multiple streams of cash flow.

**Leverage Yourself into Multiple Income Channels**

If there were two skill sets that I could get you to focus on that would be transferable to any business you do now and into the future, those would be:

1) Marketing (specifically online); and

2) Communication (speaking, selling, educating).

When you know how to market an idea online with social media, funnels, and all that razzmatazz, you will always be in demand and be able to charge small and medium businesses consulting fees to do the marketing for them.

When you are skilled at communicating with people, building rapport, selling without selling, educating or teaching, you can hire yourself out as a trainer, and teach others how to teach and speak and communicate and sell.

These two skill sets can feed you for life. When you understand marketing and funnels, you will know how to attract clients and customers to your service. *"And then He said to them, 'Follow Me, and I will make you fishers of men.'"* (Matthew 4:19 NKJV)

Business is about people. And people are engaged through the medium of communication. People will continue to buy. Why? Because we've been buying and selling since Adam and Eve. Commerce makes the world go round. So, the day we stop buying and selling is the day we stop communicating with one another, sharing and influencing each other with the richness of our differences, cultures, and ideas within the bigger cosmos of global unity...the day this stops...is the day we cease to live as human beings.

Education has become the biggest shift in opportunity for the entrepreneur. More specifically, build a business that educates a better way of doing business.

Old academic institutions just can't keep up with the pace of change in technology and learning against the barrage of free information on the internet. Real-world education is becoming privatized, and for the knowledge entrepreneur, that's a huge opportunity.

If you're struggling to come up with a business idea, get into the intellectual property business— the business of knowledge, skills, and teaching the "how."

Remember how I told you earlier that there are three types of people—1) those that do; 2) those that do it better; and 3) those who sell and teach doing it better?

Be the third type. The knowledge is already inside you; all you need is a way to get it out there.

The only reason why you haven't yet created the kind of lifestyle you're dreaming about is because someone hasn't helped you extract the value that's already inside you, or taught you how to get it out there into the world, and do it in a multitude of ways.

## Giving Back from Years of Experience

You have to write your book. Because there's a book inside you waiting to come out.

There is a level of positive energy released into the universe, marked by the signature of pure gratitude in giving.

I hated reading when I was a kid. Books were for nerds. I'm literally laughing to myself as I write these words, because I'm now the award-winning author of *The Big Shift*. I have my own book, and that's a pretty cool feeling. What's even cooler is knowing that a lot of people are learning something new from you, reconnecting the dots to that one thing that's been missing.

I hated reading so much that my dad used to hound me for not appreciating the beauty of words. Since I loved to play sports, he tried to get me to at least read the sports section of the newspaper.

That didn't work.

I still remember going with my dad to this big Swindon book store, down on Locke Road, in Tsim Sha Tsui, in Hong Kong. Dad wouldn't let me leave until I picked out a book.

So I was left alone, walking like a zombie, up and down the stacks of books that piled high to the ceiling. I started flicking through some. Here was my scientific criteria in book selection: If it was heavy, it went back on the shelf. If the words were really small, back on the shelf. If it had big words and lots of pictures, I could live with that!

The book I eventually chose was the biography of 5 times Wimbledon champion, Bjorn Borg. It had big words and lots of pictures.

I was now off the hook with Dad.

I started appreciating books much later in life because I realised I didn't know what I needed to learn, until my mentor told me to read all the best books on copywriting, and start implementing the techniques into my marketing funnels. I made over $100,000 over the next several months.

When I recently learnt how simple and easy it is to write a book, I kicked myself for not having discovered it sooner.

By the way, I'll let you in on a little secret about how I'm writing this chapter…

*…I'm speaking my book into existence.*

The technology of voice recognition is just getting better and better and better. Just open up any Google Doc document, click on "Tools" in the menu bar, and switch on "Voice Typing." Press the microphone icon once, and speak. Your words will start appearing on the screen as your book begins to unfold. And, if you've got a pretty good picture of what you want to cover in a chapter (I've already taught you how to structure your thoughts and speak fluently from my chapter on speaking.), there'd be no reason why you couldn't complete a chapter in under an hour just by speaking into the microphone.

It's not perfect yet, and you have to go back and do some editing and spell-checking, but at least it puts down your thoughts on paper without it being stuck in your head and collecting dust.

Your book is a great way to give back from your years of experience, and to leave a legacy in the world. But it's also another way that you can create content and value for your clients in the marketplace.

So, don't guard your knowledge. Write your book, teach a webinar from your book, get a speaking gig from your book, create a podcast from your book, build out a course from your book—are you getting it?

The amount of quality value you put out in the marketplace is going to build your brand, your business, your bank account, and your life.

And then you laugh.

Did you know that there is a list of bonuses that comes with your purchase of this book?

One of them is the MP3 audio version of this book. More and more people, who want to read but don't have the time, are turning to faster methods of acquiring knowledge. Now you can outsource somebody to read a book for you, and consume entire books in less than 2 hours. It's called an audiobook: You're paying somebody to read you the book, and you can just speed up the audio to get through the book in less than a couple of hours.

I used to co-lead a mastermind seminar with an awesome guy who used to read at close to 3x the speed. I mean it sounded absolutely gibberish. I asked Tom how he could even begin to decipher what he was listening to. He gave me some scientific astrophysics quantum leap theory of how your brain gets triggered in absorbing a whole lot more with speed. I didn't have the faintest idea what Tom was talking about, but I think the gist of it was that over time, your brain just gets used to the speed.

So, if you haven't got any of my bonuses yet, just head on over to www.MakeTheBigShiftBook.com, and I'll send them all to you.

Now, if you're a budding author and want to learn simple ways to get your book out, in the smoothest, fastest way possible, then go to the same website, find my contact details, and just reach out to me with a message, and I'll point you in the right direction.

## The Wealth Mindset Manifest

We live in a world where money and becoming wealthy is seen in such a negative light. We've been trained to believe that money is *the root of all evil*, and that the rich people in the world are a bunch of snobs that don't deserve their wealth, or you have to be born into money, or just be lucky enough to hit some kind of jackpot.

How often have you heard, "money doesn't grow on trees," or, "you need a good education, and a steady safe job, and you need to work 40-plus hours a week just to get by." These sayings do come from good intentions, and are meant to help us. But they also come from a state of fear and lack, which will only bring more of it.

These so-called words of wisdom have only trained your mind to settle for less, to play it safe, and have closed up your mind to the limitless opportunities out there. You have been trained to live in a world of lack and limitation, and the beliefs you have in your mind will always create the world around you.

When you continue to believe in these limiting beliefs, you will continue living a poor life, only dreaming and wishing you had more to enjoy with your family and loved ones.

And the only difference between you achieving the complete change in your life you're looking for, is to overcome what's holding you back.

For you to change the lives of other people, who do you have to change first?

This is the wealth mindset shift that I use to start my speaking engagements all around the world...and it always gets to people. I just want to make one clarification: Money itself is not evil. It is *"...the love of money that is the root of all evil."* (1 Timothy 6:10 NKJV).

It is the energy of money, or your misguided concepts of money, that really screws with you.

My money energy was programmed on dependency. I did what everyone else did: worked in a job dependent on a monthly paycheck—and for a long time, that life prescription seemed to be going well. It wasn't until the grind started to get harder each year—money was the same, my time was being tugged on more and more, and I was feeling that my own values and integrity were being sapped away—that I was slipping into the biggest self-denial and deception.

When you put a frog in a pot of cold water, then slowly turn up the heat, the frog will eventually boil itself to death, because it will learn how to adapt to the temperature increase.

I only realised this when I got out of the pot. I had to completely start over again.

For over twenty years, I had a routine. That routine was called the rat race: I woke up every morning knowing where I had to be; over half my waking hours a week were taken by the company, and then I would return home exhausted, and everything would repeat itself all over again. I'm not complaining about work, and as humans, we all should be productive. The issue is the imbalance of trade terms: Your entire livelihood and dependency is given to someone else's mercy, who is now exploiting you. It's become a poker game: accept the terms, or dare to cash in and look for something else.

I came across a Facebook post a while back, and it was a story about a big consulting guru out of New Zealand. The post was actually a *story ad* format that has become incredibly popular on Facebook. He was using his backstory and a blog-style format to promote his upcoming free webinar. The story was captivating, and it talked about the idea that if you want to succeed from where you are today, you have to *die to your old self*, rise up, and build a new version of you. The knowledge and skill set of your old self only got you so far, to a point where you are now frustrated and unfulfilled in your career choice in life. If you want something more, you need a new skill set. Your old ones have expired.

To restore, renovate, or rejuvenate anything, requires a painful and necessary process of getting rid of the old, sorting out the useful, and likely throwing a whole bunch of garbage out the window. In its place, you put in the good stuff. The laws of nature will always determine that whenever a vacuum is created, there is a universal need to fill it.

What you put in that new space is up to you.

## 20/20 Hindsight: My Final Words of Advice

So many great ideas are littered in the graveyard, which were never given the chance to bear fruit, and will never be discovered.

I *burned my boats* on June 1st, 2014, after a year of looking for a job without success. I told all my headhunters to take my name off the list: I wasn't going back. I decided to become an entrepreneur, to become among the 1% minority who are crazily courageous and ridiculed by social norms. But it was my decision, not anyone else's.

About a year later, I found myself, with my family, down in Thailand for a Mastermind event. The mastermind idea was formulated by Andrew Carnegie, and was captured in what is *the* book on self-development: Napoleon Hill's, *Think and Grow Rich*. When two experts gather together, a *third eye* appears—that is the *master mind*. Today, it has evolved into a peer-to- peer mentoring group, where two or more individuals gather together in harmony to solve major problems in business, or in anything in life.

It was at that mastermind that I *launched* myself.

Wrap yourself around successful people, and the folks who made the jump years before you did. They can give you a crystal ball of your possible future, and inspire you.

How you use your time is incredibly important. Focus on family, because you've likely got many years to catch up on. Create productive work habits in environments where you know you can excel. Eliminate the people who will waste your time or drag you back to your old self.

That's why, when I wrote *The Big Shift*, I wanted to dedicate it to you who wants more—to folks around the world who are stuck and frustrated in a job they *think* they can't leave. They have hopes and dreams for a better way but don't know how to go about getting it.

Haven't you been asking yourself *the* question for way too long without a definitive answer? ...you know what that question is.

I'm not saying that a job career is bad. But the idea of financial security, fulfillment, and work-life balance is a thing of the past.

If you're still in your job, see it from a different perspective: The company is paying you for your consultancy and expertise. Instead of considering yourself an employee, see yourself as a consultant, and the company you're working for as your major client...learn how business works so that you're ready to launch yourself. And if that makes you fulfilled, then great. The minute you're comfortable in your sense of security in a job, that's when the trouble starts.

At the end of the day, it comes down to the passion you have for what you do, the fulfillment of knowing you're living your life purpose, and the freedom of choice to decide what you want to do with your time.

But if the *job thing* is getting unbearable, stick it out long enough until you have a plan. Learn as much as you can now, while being the consultant for your company, so you can shamelessly steal your knowledge to build your own business.

My warning to you is this: Time is ticking.

The odds are stacked against you with staying in a job you absolutely love and that can give you the life balance you desire.

Prepare a plan. Plan to succeed.

I wish someone had told me that piece of advice during my last year in my job. The transition would have been a lot smoother.

What should you start a business in?

These are the biggest niches and trends you need to look into for a long-term sustainable business. Some are emerging, and some will always be a huge opportunity, and anything outside of these are likely short-term trends, up to 10 years, before they'll fizzle out: health, beauty, education, business consulting, E-commerce, storage (physical and virtual), logistics, artificial intelligence, robotics, alternative energy.

The key to any long-term business idea is the problem the solution is trying to solve. Will the problem always be there and continue to evolve into a greater and greater pain that needs to be solved?

If you can identify this, then chances are, you're onto something. Nurture it.

## Shift the Bigger Picture

No one ever just succeeds as an entrepreneur. It takes years of grinding, and trial and error, until the ingredients *click*. It takes a burning desire to do what it takes, an educational process and acquiring new skills, a positive supportive environment...and help.

The good news is, success is a learnable science.

If you've taken this book seriously, the sound bites have only triggered what is the start of your new beginning, and not the end of everything.

This is your second chance...to finally make that big shift.

I wish you every success, blessing, adventure, and sense of wonder of living out your life as it was heavenly designed.

I want to leave you with Charlie Chaplin's speech from *The Great Dictator*, one of the greatest and most inspiring ever. Filmed in 1940, it is more relevant today than when it was written.

To your journey,

**Ian D. Billingham**

*"I'm sorry, but I don't want to be an emperor. That's not my business. I don't want to rule or conquer anyone. I should like to help everyone, if possible—Jew, Gentile, black man, white. We all want to help one another. Human beings are like that. We want to live by each other's happiness, not by each other's misery. We don't want to hate and despise one another. In this world, there is room for everyone. And the good earth is rich and can provide for everyone. The way of life can be free and beautiful, but we have lost the way.*

*Greed has poisoned men's souls, has barricaded the world with hate, and has goose-stepped us into misery and bloodshed. We have developed speed, but we have shut ourselves in. Machinery that gives abundance has left us in want. Our knowledge has made us cynical. Our cleverness, hard and unkind. We think too much and feel too little. More than machinery, we need humanity. More than cleverness, we need kindness and gentleness. Without these qualities, life will be violent and all will be lost.*

*The aeroplane and the radio have brought us closer together. The very nature of these inventions cries out for the goodness in men—cries out for universal brotherhood—for the unity of us all. Even now, my voice is reaching millions throughout the world—millions of despairing men, women, and children—victims of a system that makes men torture and imprison innocent people.*

*To those who can hear me, I say, do not despair. The misery that is now upon us is but the passing of greed—the bitterness of men who fear the way of human progress. The hate of men will pass, and dictators die, and the power they took from the people will return to the people. And so long as men die, liberty will never perish.*

*Soldiers! Don't give yourselves to brutes—men who despise you, enslave you, who regiment your lives, tell you what to do, and what to think and what to feel! Who drill you, diet you, treat you like cattle, and use you as cannon fodder. Don't give yourselves to these unnatural men—machine men with machine minds and machine hearts! You are not machines! You are not cattle! You are men! You have the love of humanity in your hearts! You don't hate! Only the unloved hate—the unloved and the unnatural! Soldiers! Don't fight for slavery! Fight for liberty!*

*In the 17th Chapter of St Luke, it is written: "the Kingdom of God is within man"—not one man nor a group of men, but in all men! In you! You, the people, have the power—the power to create machines. The power to create happiness! You, the people, have the power to make this life free and beautiful, to make this life a wonderful adventure.*

*Then, in the name of democracy, let us use that power—let us all unite. Let us fight for a new world—a decent world that will give men a chance to work—that will give youth a future and old age a security. By the promise of these things, brutes have risen to power. But they lie! They do not fulfil that promise. They never will!*

*Dictators free themselves, but they enslave the people! Now, let us fight to fulfil that promise! Let us fight to free the world—to do away with national barriers—to do away with greed, with hate, and intolerance. Let us fight for a world of reason, a world where science and progress will lead to all men's happiness. Soldiers! In the name of democracy, let us all unite!"*

*The Great Dictator* (by Charlie Chaplin), 1940.

# ABOUT THE AUTHOR

Ian is a seasoned corporate executive, entrepreneur, and accomplished international speaker and trainer, with a career that spans over 27 years.

Born and raised in Hong Kong, and having lived and worked all over the world, his international corporate career has spanned multiple industries, including hotel management, sports marketing and athlete representation, and brand and consumer products marketing with some of the world's most famous brands.

Seeing how the economy is changing the paradigm of entrepreneurship and the opportunities that abound, Ian decided to leave the corporate world, back in 2013, and has started business ventures in shopping, mobile apps development, the beverage industry, digital marketing, and coaching.

One of Ian's greatest passions is in teaching and coaching entrepreneurs and seasoned business owners, on the enormous opportunities and traps in new business and wealth creation that is in front of us, following the shift into the new digital age. He shares many of his own hard lessons and experiences, and global perspective, having spoken on stages in Canada, United Kingdom, Central America, Hong Kong, Singapore, Thailand, and Australia. Today, Ian is Chief Operating Officer and private investor in an international hair and beauty company, in designing a new way of doing business.

Ian now lives in London, United Kingdom, with his wife, Susy, and kids, Michael and Yasmin, and pet pooch, Hiro.

Make sure you head over to **www.MakeTheBigShiftBook.com** to get hold of all your bonuses that Ian refers to, which come with this book.

Ian also trains small businesses and new entrepreneurs on business strategy, branding, product development, and speaking and mentoring, either in a group or on a one-on-one basis. For more details and enquiries, send him an email at the address below.

To ask Ian a question, to make a comment, or to leave him your thoughts and feedback, head over to **www.MakeTheBigShift Book.com.**

Or send him an email at: **Ready2@MakeTheBigShiftBook.com**. Ian answers every email personally.